1992

Verny

More praise from the experts for *The H.A.R.T. Program:*

"Anyone with high blood pressure *must* have a copy of *The H.A.R.T. Program.* The balanced approach in this book can empower millions of Americans to reduce and even eliminate the use of antihypertensive drugs . . . . *The H.A.R.T. Program* is essential for appropriate blood pressure control and critical to the health of the American public."
—Joe and Theresa Graedon, syndicated columnists and authors of the best-selling *People's Pharmacy* books

". . . integrates the best of ancient wisdom with the latest scientific research to give you practical, powerful tools. This book can help save your life or that of a loved one. Read it please."
—Harold H. Bloomfield, M.D., author of *Making Peace With Your Parents, Making Peace With Yourself* and *How to Survive the Loss of a Love*

". . . a state-of-the-art review of effective non-drug approaches to the treatment of hypertension. . . . A must for all patients with high blood pressure, especially those who want to eliminate or reduce drugs and their adverse side effects."
—Paul J. Rosch, M.D., F.A.C.P., Clinical Professor of Medicine in Psychiatry, New York Medical College

". . . reveals ways in which we can learn to shift our attitudes so we can find inner peace and a better balance between mind, body, and spirit."
—Gerald G. Jampolsky, M.D., author of *Love Is Letting Go of Fear*

THE H.A.R.T. PROGRAM

Lower Your Blood Pressure

Without Drugs

Dr. D. Ariel Kerman
with Richard Trubo

HarperCollins*Publishers*

The H.A.R.T. Program. Copyright © 1992 by D. Ariel Kerman. All rights reserved. Printed in the United States of America. No part of this book may be used or reproduced in any manner whatsoever without written permission except in the case of brief quotations embodied in critical articles and reviews. For information, address HarperCollins Publishers, 10 East 53rd Street, New York, New York 10022.

FIRST EDITION

Library of Congress Catalog Card Number 91-50441

ISBN 0-06-016575-8

92 93 94 95 96 AC/HC 10 9 8 7 6 5 4 3 2 1

The HART Program is dedicated to my parents, Belle and Hal Kerman, for a lifetime of love and understanding.

We are in a period of metamorphosis, a period of shedding old forms in order to manifest the highest biological and visionary ideals of the human species. That is the vocation for all of us at the turn of the twenty-first century.

—KENNETH R. PELLETIER, PH.D.
In *Longevity: Fulfilling Our Biological Potential*

Contents

Author's Note

I FIRST BECAME aware of stress- and lifestyle-related disorders as major contributors to psychological and physiological disorders in modern society during graduate studies at the University of Chicago. It was then that I made the commitment to identify, develop, and mainstream cost-effective, noninvasive solutions to hypertension and other major health problems. Since then, in more than a decade of working as a clinician, psychotherapist, researcher, and organizational consultant, my primary goal has been to assist my patients and clients in taking a solution-based approach to setting and achieving health and life outcomes that are of high importance to them. Many of the individuals discover that high blood pressure and other problems can be opportunities for improving their health.

The HART Program is a product of this clinical work, research, and program development. It is the first time a comprehensive, step-by-step, self-directed biobehavioral program for normalizing blood pressure has been made available in book form. This program has been developed concurrently with the creation of the HART Institute, founded as a vehicle to provide comprehensive programs for health enhancement and longevity.

A major benefit of the program described in this book, in addition to lowering blood pressure and reducing or eliminating the need for medication, is that most participants experience being more in control of life stress and feeling more energetic, happier, more peaceful, rested, and productive.

Health and happiness are your birthright. It is my hope that this book assists you in attaining that which is rightfully yours.

We at the HART Institute would enjoy hearing from you: 645 N. Michigan Ave., Suite 800, Chicago, IL 60611.

D. ARIEL KERMAN, PH.D.
Director, HART Institute

Acknowledgments

THE SHARED VISION and support of many contributed to making this book a reality. In the decade I have been engaged in the clinical work, research, and writing that led to the HART Program, the dedication of my patients has been a continuing source of inspiration. Warm acknowledgment is due to these individuals who, by actively assuming responsibility for their health, are helping to bring in a new era in health care. Many participants*—executives and professionals from major corporations and organizations, homemakers, and health care providers—generously gave time to share their experiences for this book.

Doctoral work with Patricia A. Norris, Ph.D., Clinical Director, and Steven L. Fahrion, Ph.D., Director of Research at the Menninger Foundation Voluntary Controls Program, my collaborators in clinical research and on the first *HART Clinical Manual for the Biobehavioral Treatment of High Blood Pressure* (1984), was integral to the process that led to the development of this book. I am deeply appreciative of their wise counsel and excellence as mentors. I wish to further express my appreciation to Elmer Green, Ph.D., Director; and Alyse Green, M.A., Psychophysiological Therapist at the Menninger Foundation Voluntary Controls Program.

Significant support for the research which contributed to developing the HART Program was provided by the University of Illinois at Chicago School of Public Health and my colleagues at the University. I am grateful to the School of Public Health for producing the video documentary on the HART Program and for granting permission for use of material from the documentary in this work.

I especially want to thank Lyndon Babcock, Ph.D., Professor of Public Health, Environmental Engineering and Geography, who served as head of my research surveillance committee, faculty sponsor, co-author of the documentary, and reviewer of this manuscript. Others who contributed to the documentary were Edward A. Lichter, M.D., Professor of General Internal Medicine at the University of Illinois, Harold Spies, M.D., Medical Director at Amoco, and Alfred Klinger, M.D., Assistant Professor of Preventive Medicine at Rush Presbyterian St. Luke's Medical Center, Michael Brown, and Deborah Regan.

---

* Throughout this book, the names of participants have been changed to respect their privacy.

Charles A. Warren, Ph.D., Assistant Professor of Environmental and Occupational Health Sciences at the University of Illinois, brought considerable clinical insight and expertise to the research, and generously made his psychophysiological laboratory available. Joseph L. Levin, Ed.D., Associate Professor of Community Health Sciences, and Victoria W. Persky, M.D., Associate Professor of Epidemiology and Biostatistics, gave valued support.

Charles E. Thompson, M.D., a member of the Illinois Governor's Advisory Board on Hypertension, served as Medical Director during the course of the study. Virginia Swan, Ph.D., provided a context for the clinical delivery of the program. Laury Levy and Sandy Pessman of *Crain's Chicago Business*, helped the HART Program reach the corporate and professional world through the article, "Mind Over Body Masters Hypertension." Karyl Kinsey, Ph.D., provided significant editorial assistance at key points in the development of this work. Richard Stanton, Ph.D., Terry Daunter, Ph.D., and Carol Barrett, Ph.D., critically reviewed the research and encouraged me to proceed with a popular book.

One of the signs of true contributors and visionaries is their capacity to inspire, inform, and empower others to bring about needed personal and social transformation. I especially wish to acknowledge Tom Ferguson, M.D., founding editor of *Medical Self-Care* and one of the foremost advocates of medical self-help, for reviewing the manuscript and writing the Foreword to this book. Kenneth Pelletier, Ph.D., of Stanford University, whose landmark works helped bring to national attention the need to meet the challenge of stress- and lifestyle-related disorders, was instrumental in my professional commitment to this area and was an early supporter of this book. Norman Cousins also reviewed my work and encouraged me to go forward with this book. I also wish to thank Dean Ornish, M.D., clinician, researcher and author, whose studies have demonstrated that heart disease can be reversed through lifestyle change, for his support and endorsement of the program.

Many dedicated clinicians, researchers, and writers have contributed to our knowledge of the treatment and prevention of high blood pressure and other stress- and lifestyle-related disorders. Among those whose work has been an important influence upon this book are Jeremiah Stamler, M.D.; Rose Stamler, M.A.; Norman Kaplan, M.D.; Chandra Patel, M.D.; Barbara Brown, Ph.D.; Hans Selye, M.D.; Rene Dubois, M.D.; Robert Eliot, M.D.; Eric Peper, Ph.D.; Herbert Benson, M.D.; Kenneth Cooper, M.D.; David Sobel, M.D.; Jonathan Smith, Ph.D.; Blair Justice, Ph.D.; Richard Shames, M.D.; and Pir Vilayat Kahn.

The photographs in the text, which express not only precision in technique but the inner experience of relaxing deeply, are the result of the work of Belle Kerman, architectural designer, and Clyde Okita, photojournalist. Steve Quick, a jewelry designer, gave of his time to demonstrate the skills of the program.

I was fortunate in choosing Richard Trubo as my collaborator. The book benefited from Richard's wealth of knowledge and previous writings on managing chronic diseases.

That this comprehensive guide is written is largely due to the vision and belief in the work by Carol Cohen, my publisher at HarperCollins; and Andrea Sargent, my editor at HarperCollins, who fine-tuned the text.

Lois Shapiro, associate publisher of Basic Books, and Joel Belsky, my "sunrise hiking partners" at Rancho La Puerta, proposed that I write a book on the HART Program, and brought my proposal to HarperCollins. I consider them godparents of the book. I also wish to thank Deborah Szekely, co-founder of Rancho La Puerta.

I also wish to express my appreciation to Martha Faulhaber, Clarence Klingert, James Swann, Beatrice Briggs, Lois Dobry, Malcolm Weiskopf, Evangeline Bay, and Kathleen Mathis, for providing input to the work in progress; John and Tom Frangias, Kahlil, Jed Katch, Ph.D., Marnell Scott and Vi Uretz for giving of their time; David Harris, Mary Thompson, Michael Castleman, and Beverly Merz for networking on behalf of the book; E. Leonard Rubin and Leon M. Despres for their wise counsel; Elee Purry for the care of my household; and Lee Botts for a sanctuary in which to write.

The support and caring of my parents, Belle and Hal Kerman, to whom this book is dedicated, and my sister, Shani Kerman, made working on the book possible. I wish to thank my family and friends for their patience, understanding, and especially for their presence, which makes this a more loving world in which to live.

Those whose lives touch ours are diamonds in the constellation of our lives.

Foreword

YOU HAVE HIGH blood pressure, and you're determined to do everything you can to bring it down to normal.

If you are now taking drugs to bring your pressure down, you'd like to get off them altogether—or at least reduce their use to an absolute minimum. If you haven't yet started taking anti-hypertension drugs, you'd like to avoid them.

This book will help you do exactly that.

The HART Program is the most comprehensive guide currently available to bringing your blood pressure back to normal using biobehavioral, self-care, non-drug methods. It provides a step-by-step set of guidelines for using the latest scientific principles to allow you to control your blood pressure. Indeed, this book covers virtually everything known to science that you can do to bring your blood pressure down without drugs.

You may have sought out this book because you have experienced one or more of the unpleasant side effects of antihypertensive drugs—dry mouth, dizziness, cramps, sexual dysfunction, or other known effects. If so, you are not alone. The side effects of these drugs are all too common and all too difficult to manage. Physicians have a difficult time convincing their patients to take these drugs even where they are truly needed.

Not many of us would choose to take a powerful chemical when safer treatments are available. Treatment with high blood pressure drugs is not always simple or straightforward. You may develop tolerance for one or more of these drugs and thus require a larger dose. You may have to change to another drug, or to a combination of drugs—and with every change, you will face the renewed risk of side effects.

Thus most conscientious physicians today encourage their patients to control their blood pressure without drugs if at all possible, reserving pharmacological treatment as a last resort for those cases which cannot be controlled by the methods described in this book.

With the publication of *The HART Program*, the non-drug treatment of high blood pressure has become much easier than ever before. Among those who have completed the program on which this book is based, the results are spectacular indeed: nine out of ten participants were able to lower their blood pressure. Seven out of ten were able to withdraw from their high blood pressure drugs altogether. Some took only a few weeks. Some took several months. Others have been able to reduce their dose of drugs to an absolute minimum. You can do the same.

The self-management of high blood pressure—and other health conditions—is the way of the future. Scientific evidence makes it clear that, while drugs can indeed help lower high blood pressure, they should only be used as a last resort—to treat those cases that can not be managed by self-care measures.

This shift toward self-care is a part of a greater historical trend: health power is beginning to move out of our doctors' offices, clinics, and hospitals. It is moving into our homes, our schools, and the places in which we work. We are realizing that there is more and more we can all do to prevent illness and to manage health problems.

To keep pace with this important shift in responsibility, each of us needs to master new health skills. We need to keep ourselves up to date on the latest discoveries about stress, diet, fitness, the importance of support, and other self-care priorities. Plus, we must learn to work with health professionals as informed, health-active consumers, not as passive patients.

We are accepting the fact that these self-help measures should be our first line of defense in our battle for good health. Nowhere is this more true than in managing high blood pressure.

The new health care system of the 1990's and beyond will accept the fact that the major determinants of health, fitness, and longevity will be the personal choices made by each individual. *The HART Program: Lower Your Blood Pressure without Drugs* is about those choices.

Dr. Kerman is a pioneering leader and expert in the patient-centered control of high blood pressure. She integrates a broad scientific knowledge of behavioral medicine, blood pressure, and cardiovascular health with sound clinical methods to help you accomplish desired personal change. Her book will provide you with a wide range of information, alternatives, options, and resources.

I would encourage you to begin with the techniques that interest you most. Some people prefer to begin with relaxation and stress management. Others choose to start with dietary change or exercise. Eventually, you may choose to combine several of these approaches. The best path for you is the one that takes account of your own special background, preferences, and interests. By committing yourself to doing all you can to reduce or eliminate your need for medication, you will be taking a giant step in the direction of self-responsibility for your own health.

My expectation is that the benefits of this program will go far beyond the ability to control your blood pressure. It will help put control into your own hands. It will make you more autonomous, more responsible. It will give you the tools and skills you will be able to use not only to control your blood pressure, but many other areas of your life.

The HART Program will help you develop your own tailor-made self-care program for managing your high blood pressure. This is a healthy, empowering, constructive program that will yield great benefits in all parts of your life.

Tom Ferguson, M.D.
Graduate, Yale Medical School
Founding Editor, *Medical Self-Care*

PART I

Lowering Your Blood Pressure with HART: Background and Rationale

CHAPTER 1

Lowering Your Blood Pressure With HART

I wanted to control my blood pressure and do it without *drugs. I'm the kind of person who likes to feel in control of the situation and not be dependent on something on the outside to care for my body. So HART fit in with my general view of the world. I think people should have some control over their own health.*

—TODD
Insurance executive
HART participant

APPROXIMATELY ONE OUT of every three adults—or 60 million Americans—have high blood pressure or *hypertension*. Until recently, antihypertensive medication has been the mainstay of high blood pressure treatment. Today, however, our nation is in the midst of a healthy revolution regarding the treatment of high blood pressure. More than ever before, leading experts in hypertension are emphasizing the importance of nondrug methods for treating high blood pressure.

The Joint National Committee on Detection, Evaluation and Treatment of High Blood Pressure has been at the forefront of the present shift in thinking. This policymaking panel, composed of leading hypertension experts, has called for nondrug lifestyle interventions as the *front line* treatment for individuals with mild hypertension. Over half of all people with high blood pressure are in this category. Equally important, the joint committee has recommended that once high blood pressure is under control, nonpharmacological methods should be used by **all** hypertensives to reduce their medication needs and, when possible, elimiate medications entirely.

HART—Hypertension, Autonomic, Relaxation Treatment—is a breakthrough biobehavioral and lifestyle program designed to lower high blood pressure and eliminate the need for antihypertensive medication. According to *Harrison's Principles of Internal Medicine*, elevated arterial pressure is the most important public health problem in developed countries, being common, asymptomatic, readily detectable, usually easily treatable, and often leading to lethal complications if left untreated. Nonpharmacological treatment programs such as HART are part of the new paradigm in healthcare that places cost-effective resources for self-care in the hands of those who need them.

The objective of the HART Program is to provide you with the information and step-by-step guidelines you need to successfully reach your blood pressure goals.

The biobehavioral core of the HART Program consists of deep psychophysiological relaxation training and stress management assisted by temperature feedback. It is based on a protocol initially developed and tested at the Menninger Foundation's Voluntary Controls program which, in over a decade of clinical use, has shown itself to be a highly effective method for normalizing blood pressure and thus eliminating the need for medication. Hypertension—like 50 to 80 percent of all physical and psychological illnesses—is stress-related. A large majority of individuals reach their blood pressure goals through biobehavioral

---

The HART Program is a cost-effective, noninvasive treatment approach to the costly personal and national health problem of high blood pressure. Current healthcare costs in the United States have soared to $606 billion, up from $230 billion just a decade ago. Costs are approaching $2 billion a day. If trends continue, these costs are projected to reach $1.5 trillion by the end of the 1990s.

Costs for hypertension were $13.7 billion in 1991, or about $37 million a day. That figure includes $4 billion for hospitalization, nearly $3 billion for antihypertensive medication, and over $2 billion in lost workdays. However, when you consider that approximately 60 million of the 68 million Americans with CVD have high blood pressure, which is a major contributing cause of cardiovascular disease, then the actual human and economic costs of high blood pressure are substantially higher.

The cost of treating cardiovascular disease in 1991 in the U.S. reached $101.3 billion dollars, including doctor fees, nursing services, the cost of medication, nursing home care, and loss of productivity.

With skyrocketing healthcare costs becoming increasingly burdensome for individuals and businesses, and with millions of Americans uninsured, cost-effective healthcare options need to be an important individual and national priority if our country is to be able to offer quality healthcare to all its citizens.

methods alone. Biobehavioral treatment has resulted in as many as seven of ten patients normalizing their blood pressure and completely eliminating their need for medications.

If your objectives are to lower your blood pressure and reduce your overall cardiovascular risk, it makes sense to incorporate a fuller range of healthy lifestyle choices into your personal program. In addition to stress management, approaches like adopting healthier eating habits, increasing exercise, shedding excess pounds, and ceasing smoking can all contribute to lower blood pressure and greater cardiovascular health.

This book, therefore, provides guidelines for using a broad spectrum of nonpharmacological or nondrug methods that will assist you in both attaining your blood pressure objectives and protecting and improving your cardiovascular health. The benefits of taking charge of your blood pressure are a longer, healthier, happier life.

THE ORIGINS OF THE HART PROGRAM

In 1984, I began conducting research on the biobehavioral treatment of high blood pressure. My initial study was undertaken as part of a research associateship at the University of Illinois School of Public Health, in association with Dr. Patricia Norris and Dr. Steven Fahrion, clinical director and director of research of the Menninger Voluntary Controls program and Dr. Charles Warren, associate professor at the University of Illinois. My goal was to test whether this basic biobehavioral approach would be effective as a more largely home-based program of self-care that would minimize the need for direct clinical assistance.

The results, presented at both the National Conference on High Blood Pressure Control and at the Association for Applied Psychophysiology and Biofeedback, were promising. My patients in the largely home-based group, who participated in less than half the standard number of clinic sessions, did just as well in reducing their blood pressure and their need for medication as those in the more standard, clinically-intensive program.

The HART Clinical Manual for the Biobehavioral Treatment of High Blood Pressure: A Systematic Cost-Effective Program to Normalize Blood Pressure and Become Medication-Free, which I wrote in collaboration with Drs. Norris and Fahrion, was developed in the course of this study. It was the first detailed guide to the HART Program. My patients in the program found the manual a valuable guide for home practice, and there was considerable demand for the text from professionals. I recognized that a more comprehensive book was needed to serve as a resource for individuals who wanted to use a nonpharmacological approach in taking control of their own blood pressure. The result is *The HART Program,* the book you now hold in your hands.

WILL THE HART PROGRAM WORK FOR YOU?

If you and I were meeting together, what would you want to know? My patients are most interested in the track record for biobehavioral treatment, who this approach has been effective for, whether it will work for them, and what they need to do in order to succeed.

The basic biobehavioral protocol on which this program is based actually has more than a fifteen-year track record of clinical use, dating back to its origins at the Menninger Foundation. It has been effective for young and old; for individuals with mild, moderate, and even severe high blood pressure; for those in whom hypertension has only recently been diagnosed; and for persons who have had high blood pressure and have been on antihypertensive medications for several decades. Given this record, the likelihood of the HART Program working for you, too, is excellent.

As a clinician, I have worked with individuals from their early twenties through their eighties and seen them regain control over their blood pressure, while either completely eliminating or substantially reducing their need for medication. The basic program has been successful for almost everyone.

Let me describe for you a long-term study on the biobehavioral treatment of high blood pressure on which the HART Program is based. It was conducted at the Menninger Foundation by Dr. Elmer Green, Dr. Fahrion, and Dr. Norris, and involved 60 patients with high blood pressure, 42 of whom entered the study on antihypertensive medications. These individuals went through a program consisting of a rationale for how the program worked, training in the use of temperature feedback to reduce overactivation of the sympathetic branch of the autonomic nervous system and techniques for reducing chronic muscle tension, establishing correct breathing patterns, managing stress, and learning how to monitor their blood pressure at home.

The study found that about 90 percent of the patients achieved significant reductions in their systolic and diastolic blood pressure, as well as declines in their antihypertensive medication use. Of those patients who entered biobehavioral treatment on medications:

69 percent were able to eliminate their medication entirely while reducing blood pressure by 15/10 mm of mercury (Hg).

21 percent, while not withdrawing from medication completely, had their dosages cut approximately in half, and lowered their blood pressure by 18/10 mm Hg.

Only 10 percent of the patients showed no improvement in either blood pressure or medication requirements. This group included individuals who did not regularly practice the techniques.

Similar results were found for nonmedicated patients.

The basic techniques of biobehavioral treatment are sufficiently straightforward that nearly everyone who learns and practices them achieves results. An important advantage of biobehavioral treatment is that the improvements you achieve tend to persist. Not only does blood pressure decline and stabilize at a normal level, but for many people, this outcome is maintained over time. According to researchers at the Voluntary Controls program at the Menninger Foundation, the results of biobehavioral therapy for many participants have been sustained for as long as nine years. Of equal significance, once individuals have succeeded in lowering their blood pressure, they have the skills and resources to bring it down once again if they experience later increases in blood pressure.

Two important cautions are necessary. **First, this program is intended only for persons who have been diagnosed with *essential* or primary hypertension,** which means that there is no known medical cause for their high blood pressure. About 95 percent of all individuals with hypertension fall into this category. The remaining five percent of patients have *secondary* hypertension, which is high blood pressure caused by an identifiable medical condition such as kidney disease or a benign tumor of the adrenal glands; in these cases, other treatments are necessary. In this book, the term *high blood pressure* or *hypertension* refers to essential hypertension unless otherwise indicated. If you are uncertain about your own diagnosis, check with your doctor.

Second, if you are on medications when you start this program, consult your physician before beginning the program, and keep him or her informed of your progress. **Make no changes in your medication without your doctor's approval and supervision.** Discontinuing your medication abruptly can be hazardous to your health. Please work closely with your physician for any medication changes.

WHAT DOES THE PROGRAM INVOLVE?

Your success in using the biobehavioral program to reach your blood pressure goals depends on regular practice of feedback-assisted, deep psychophysiological relaxation for 15 minutes twice daily, using a series of straightforward, self-regulatory skills that form the core of the program. In addition, you will be asked to take and record your blood pressure, pulse, and body peripheral temperature (an objective indicator of relaxation) before and after your relaxation practice to chart your progress. Once you have learned these skills, you will be asked to apply them—along with stress management—in your daily life, using a strategy called Constant Instant Practice.

WHEN WILL YOU SEE RESULTS?

How soon can you expect to see results with the HART Program? Many participants begin to experience improvements almost immediately. Following your initial relaxation sessions, you will very likely see measurable declines in blood pressure readings. The time needed to attain longer-term blood pressure goals can vary. Some patients have lowered their blood pressure and eliminated medications in as little as five weeks; however, the average participant is able to eliminate medications within 20 weeks after beginning treatment. However long it takes, I generally recommend that my patients continue their deep psychophysiological relaxation and stress management practice for several months after they have attained the results they want, in order to stabilize their improvements over the long term, and that they resume practice during particularly stressful times or if they notice increases in their blood pressure.

When you consider that many individuals who choose biobehavioral treatment have been on antihypertensive medication for two to three decades, 20 weeks is a relatively brief period to regain self-regulatory control of blood pressure. For those who have been diagnosed more recently, the time they invest in this program may prevent them from ever starting on medication or needing it over the long term. The 20-week average is for individuals whose program emphasized primarily biobehavioral techniques without other lifestyle changes; if you choose instead a more comprehensive nonpharmacological approach like the one detailed in this book, you may achieve your blood pressure objectives more rapidly. I recommend, however, that you continue with the full 20 weeks of the program in the interest of maintaining long-term results.

By practicing the biobehavioral techniques and incorporating the lifestyle changes of the HART Program, you will begin to achieve and gradually maintain a lower, healthier blood pressure without—or with substantially less—reliance on medication. As Dr. Elmer Green, developer of the original biobehavioral protocol at the Menninger Foundation, says most encouragingly, "Those who persist, succeed."

SETTING YOURSELF UP TO SUCCEED

This book is designed as a self-care guide. It includes all the information you need to successfully implement your own program to normalize your blood pressure. If, however, you feel you would benefit from more personalized clinical support, I encourage you to work with a clinician or therapist who has a background in relaxation, stress management, biofeedback training, and lifestyle change. While working with a clinician is certainly not necessary, many individuals find that personalized guidance contributes to their success and enjoyment. At the HART Institute, we offer ongoing as well as intensive programs. Some individuals accomplish their personal health objectives independently with little external structure; others do much better with some assistance. If you think you are more likely to successfully follow through with this program with the support of a clinician, then it makes good sense to find a competent, experienced, clinician to help you achieve important health goals. Know yourself and set yourself up to succeed.

I personally think that some support and encouragement helps individuals stay with the program over time. Your physician or other health-care provider, family members, or a good friend can all be important sources of support.

To get started in the HART Program, you will want to have on hand the following equipment, which is discussed in more detail later in the book: a blood pressure measurement instrument, a few small room temperature thermometers, or another feedback device, audiotapes and a recorder, and a watch. You will also need copies of the logs which are found in Appendix II at the back of this book.

The sooner you get started with the program, the more rapidly you will see results. If you want to begin the biobehavioral program right away, go directly to Part II, Chapter 6 to learn the self-monitoring skills, and then move on to the biobehavioral techniques beginning in Chapter 7. If you choose this approach, however, I recommend that you go back and read the introductory chapters once you have launched your program.

CHAPTER · 2

Case Studies: Why Participants Choose HART

FOR MANY INDIVIDUALS, the biobehavioral components of the HART Program have been the "missing link" that has enabled them to normalize their blood pressure and eliminate or significantly reduce their need for antihypertensive medication. Many entered the HART Program already aware of the importance of diet and exercise in managing their hypertension; however, that hadn't been enough to normalize their blood pressure and eliminate medications. For the following individuals, the HART Program made the difference.

EDWARD: CORPORATE VICE-PRESIDENT

When Edward, a husband and father of three, began the HART Program, he was taking a diuretic and beta-blocker three times a day to control his blood pressure. As a vital, self-assured, 45-year-old financial company vice-president, he keenly understood the implications of high blood pressure for health and longevity, and was committed to taking charge of his own health.

There was a history of hypertension on his mother's side of the family. Edward's grandmother had died of a stroke, and his mother and sister both had high blood pressure. This family history predisposed him to developing hypertension as well.

Even though Edward walked regularly and tried to watch what he ate, his work responsibilities and travel schedule sometimes made it difficult for him to exercise and control his meals. Stress was another factor in Edward's life. As an accomplished executive working for a high-performance company, he necessarily had high objectives for himself and his staff. His high blood pressure was diagnosed at age 18, and when he was 32, his doctor placed him on medications.

What was Edward's motivation for starting the HART Program? Edward says:

> When I first started taking medication, it wasn't any big deal. But as I went on, I found that medications didn't always work. My system seemed to

become immune, and I had to keep changing medications periodically. I also began to read more about side effects. I felt after being on hypertensive medication for thirteen or fourteen years that I didn't want to do it anymore. My objective was really to get off medications.

Even with medication, Edward's initial blood pressure readings were quite high. When he started the HART Program, his blood pressure was 165/100. Soon after beginning the program, Edward saw the results of his relaxation practice.

I experienced improvements almost immediately. It took only a few sessions to bring my blood pressure down to near-normal ranges. I was very excited about it. The relaxation exercises in particular gave me a real sense of my body. After a few sessions, I could easily determine if I was under stress and could get myself to relax.

That was only the beginning, however. When Edward showed his physician his blood pressure records, his doctor was very supportive. "He was delighted I would make the effort," says Edward. "I would show him the results and tell him I was probably ready for a medication reduction, and he was very cooperative."

Edward's doctor reduced Edward's medication during the fourth and sixth weeks of the program. During week nine, the doctor took Edward off one of the two drugs he had been taking. Five weeks later, Edward was taken off all medication. Just fourteen weeks after beginning the HART Program, he was no longer taking any medication, and his blood pressure was 125/83 mm Hg—well below the 140/90 level at which individuals are considered hypertensive. He maintained his average blood pressure reading for the last four weeks of the program at 124/80.

After stabilizing his blood pressure within normal range, Edward no longer needed to practice regular deep relaxation twice a day. However, he still used the stress management techniques when he needed them, contributing to his long-term, positive results in the program. "I run into stressful situations all day long," says Edward. "I think about them now, and I am able to stop and relax."

While Edward's work responsibilities have markedly increased since he completed the HART Program three years ago, his blood pressure is still normal. In addition, he continues to be free from the multiple medications he used to rely on to control his hypertension.

TODD: INSURANCE EXECUTIVE

Todd is a trim 35-year-old who creates insurance programs for corporations. Todd says he thrives on challenge, considering himself "competitive, ambitious, and assertive, with a desire to be number one."

When Todd entered the HART Program, he was at his ideal weight, exercised regularly, and watched what he ate. Even so, at age 35, he was taking three different antihypertensive medications to keep his blood pressure under control.

Initially, Todd was skeptical about whether the program would work for him. However, he felt "it made sense that the reason I had the blood pressure problem was because of some internal inability to control my tension. And if I could learn ways to do that, I could control my blood pressure. It wasn't anything that was organically wrong with me."

Todd's family had a history of hypertension. His grandfather had died of a stroke and his mother had died of a heart attack, both in their seventies. Todd had been diagnosed as having high blood pressure at age 22. His twin brother also had hypertension. And although his doctor had adjusted his medication dosage to eliminate the headaches he had initially experienced with the drug, Todd didn't like being reliant on a pill.

"No one, I think, wants to be on medication if they can avoid it," said Todd. "It's just a hassle, and at my young age, I felt even more hampered by always having to have a supply of drugs.

"I wanted to control my blood pressure and do it **without** drugs. I'm the kind of person who likes to feel in control of the situation and not be dependent on something on the outside to care for my body. So HART fit in with my general view of the world. I think people should have some control over their own health."

Todd began practicing the relaxation techniques "religiously," as he describes it, and learned to modify his reaction to stress. As that occurred, his doctor gradually reduced his medications, and after five weeks, Todd was taken off drugs completely. Even though he stopped taking antihypertensive drugs, his blood pressure remained stable—126/73 on medication, and 122/75 once they were eliminated.

Although Todd achieved rapid results, he continued with his relaxation practice twice a day, and stress management for a few additional months. As a result, he further stabilized his blood pressure and increased his probability of staying normotensive and medication-free over the long term.

When I asked Todd to describe the program's primary effects, he responded, "It would be the awareness of what causes my blood pressure to rise, and the knowledge that I can use nonchemical methods to control it."

At one-, three-, and five-year followups, Todd's blood pressure remained normal without any antihypertensive drugs. He continues to take his own blood pressure at least once a month, and at last report, it was 135/78. He has successfully integrated the stress-management skills into his daily life and continues to use them.

"I check things out from time to time," says Todd, "and if I feel myself getting tense, I'll try one of the relaxation techniques. As I start to breathe more deeply, I'll check out what factors might be causing the stress. The program has allowed me to be more effective in my work, while maintaining my blood pressure where I want it to be."

HELEN: RETIRED SOCIAL WORKER

Helen, an engaging woman who had enjoyed a long and productive career as a social worker, entered the HART Program at age 74 with a clear determination to regain control of her blood pressure.

Helen had started taking antihypertensive medication at age 62, and when she began HART more than a decade later, her blood pressure was 147/80 on twice-a-day diuretic therapy. She enthusiastically practiced feedback-assisted relaxation and stress management. "As a social worker, I had always heard about psychosomatic illness, and that a lot of symptoms were associated with your emotions," she said. "And I thought it was true that you can calm yourself down."

Helen's blood pressure began to fall. Even so, her physician was initially slow to reduce her medications, despite the combined evidence of both her home blood pressure records and clinical measurements well below her initial readings. With time, however, her doctor cut her diuretic intake to once a day. Then, as her blood pressure dropped even further, he directed her to stop taking the medication completely.

Helen's blood pressure stayed within normal levels (about 133/68) without antihypertensive medication even during painful surgery three years after her participation in the program.

MICHAEL: BANK VICE-PRESIDENT

Michael, a distinguished bank vice-president and committed family man in his early fifties, entered the HART Program in order to find a way to manage his blood pressure without medication.

Michael's cardiologist was having difficulty keeping his potassium level in balance. The antihypertensive medication caused Michael to feel extremely fatigued, and he was concerned about the long-term effects of the medication. "I got into the program because the drug I was prescribed was very powerful and I didn't know what the effects would be over a period of years," he said.

By practicing the techniques of the program, Michael became aware of how he was responding to work-related stress and its effect upon his blood pressure. "There is a lot of stress and pressure, but I really wasn't too aware of it," he told me. "However, looking back, I would tend to tense up and it would cause difficulties for me."

When I introduced Michael to the relaxation techniques, he noted there was more to relaxation than he expected. "I, like many others, really believed that relaxation was watching television or being entertained or possibly playing golf or something like that," he said. "I think that many of us do subconsciously have stress and anxiety—things that are really bothering us. I learned that to really relax, you need to concentrate on relaxation, and some of the techniques I learned through the program enabled me to *really* relax. And there is a real difference."

During the course of the program, as Michael's doctor gradually took him off all antihypertensive medications, his blood pressure remained stable at about 124/93, then decreased to 125/89 once medications were completely eliminated.

"I learned quite a bit about blood pressure, and how to control stress," said Michael.

> I also learned a lot about myself. The program allowed me to step back and see what happens under stressful conditions—the pressure of sales and that kind of thing. I became more efficient and effective by learning how to control my emotions and deal with stress. The program gave me 25 to 30 percent more energy and pep. I've made some changes I will always think about.

ALAN: REAL ESTATE DEVELOPER

Alan, a robust man in his fifties and a successful real estate developer, was diagnosed as having borderline high blood pressure for 12 years before he entered the HART Program. He tried to normalize his hypertension through salt restriction, diet, and exercise, but still needed medications to control his blood pressure.

Alan's father, who had experienced his first heart attack at age 58, died of heart problems at age 64. Alan's mother, who had a history of high blood pressure, died of congestive heart failure following a bypass operation. During his parents' illnesses, Alan became informed about hypertension and cardiovascular disease, and had become more vigilant about his own self-care.

A few months after Alan began taking an antihypertensive drug called Tenormin, he started experiencing what he called "a deadening of emotion or motivation. The drug works on your heart, and as it slows your heart rate down, after a while you slow down."

Alan acknowledged that before finally going off the drug, he wasn't as excitable, reactive, volatile, and angry as he had been. "Now, however, I control those emotions in other ways," he said. "From the moment I started the HART Program, I could see slow steady improvement in my blood pressure. I told the doctor that the program seemed to be working and I would like to try it without the medication. I haven't gotten back on it since."

About a year after he completed the program, Alan had a stress test. He was pleased that his blood pressure was in a normal range and it stayed there throughout the test.

CHAPTER · 3

Mind, Body, and Blood Pressure

*The greatest force in the human body is the natural drive of
the body to heal itself—but that force is not independent of
the belief system, which can translate expectations into physiological change. Nothing is more wondrous about the fifteen
billion neurons in the human brain than their ability to
convert thoughts, hopes, ideas, and attitudes into chemical
substances. Everything begins, therefore, with belief. What we
believe is the most powerful option of all.*

—NORMAN COUSINS

YOUR BLOOD PRESSURE plays an important role in your health and well-
being. Let's take a brief, simplified look at what is occurring within your
body when you have high blood pressure. While it is not necessary to
have an in-depth understanding, some background will enable you to
more easily comprehend how you can regain control of your blood
pressure. In addition, let's look at the connection between the mind and
body in controlling hypertension.

WHAT IS BLOOD PRESSURE AND HOW DOES IT BECOME HIGH?

By definition, blood pressure is the force your blood exerts upon the
blood vessel walls as it travels through your body's arterial system. Medical textbooks state that blood pressure is equivalent to cardiac output
times total systemic peripheral resistance. In layperson's terms, this
means the relationship of the amount of blood pumped by the heart
(cardiac output) to the overall tightness within your blood vessels (total
systemic peripheral resistance).

When your doctor takes your blood pressure reading, he or she as-
certains two numbers. First, as your heart contracts or beats, the pressure on your arterial walls is measured: this is called the *systolic* pressure.

16

Then, when your heart relaxes or rests between contractions, the pressure on the arterial walls—your *diastolic* pressure—is determined. Your systolic pressure is the larger of the two numbers because it is a measurement of the greatest pressure that occurs against the vessel walls; by contrast, the diastolic pressure is a reflection of the lowest pressure on your blood vessel walls.

As you probably already know, your blood pressure is recorded in fraction form, with your systolic pressure on top and your diastolic pressure on the bottom. Thus, a blood pressure reading of 135/80, for example, means you have a systolic pressure of 135, and a diastolic pressure of 80. The numbers themselves refer to millimeters of mercury (mm Hg) that are displaced when the reading is taken.

As pressure is generated by each successive beat of your heart, it propels oxygenated, nutrient-rich blood to every cell, tissue, and organ in your body. When conditions and demands upon your body routinely change, your blood pressure automatically changes in order to provide the body with a sufficient supply of blood. For example, you require less oxygen and fewer nutrients while at rest than during physical exercise, or when you are relaxed rather than while feeling stressed.

Your heart is at the center of this entire process. It is a four-chambered muscle about the size of both of your fists, filled with crimson fluid. It beats about 100,000 times day, during which it pumps about 40,000 gallons of blood throughout your body.

To more vividly and tangibly picture your heart and vasculature, imagine that your fists are your heart. Interlace your fists and place them on your chest over your actual heart. A little more than once a second, squeeze your fists together, representing your heart as it contracts and responds to instructions communicated by the brain through electrical impulses. Each time your fists contract, picture about two ounces of fluid being propelled into your aorta (the large blood vessel attached to your heart muscle) and then making its way into your larger vascular system.

Next, imagine two blood vessels that are like flexible rubbery tubes about the width of a soda straw. These represent your coronary arteries, which branch out above your heart like a crown. Your red blood cells make their way through these arteries and into the intricate network of the circulatory system, dividing into smaller arterioles that in turn connect with the smallest vessels, the capillaries, which are only a fraction as thick as a human hair. The capillaries bring blood directly to the organ tissues.

The blood picks up tissue waste products and carbon dioxide, and returns them through the veins to the right side of the heart, which then pumps them through the lungs. In the lungs, the blood exchanges carbon dioxide for a fresh supply of oxygen. Meanwhile, other waste products are filtered out by the kidneys, after which cleansed blood returns to the heart's left ventricle (the heart's main pumping chamber). At this point, reoxygenated blood leaves the heart again to supply the needs of the entire body.

This circulating blood has been compared to an internal sea. It travels through a network of blood vessels that, if stretched end to end, would extend for 60,000 miles! It is amazing that a muscle about double the size of your fist can pump blood through a vascular network more than twice as large as the circumference of the earth. Yet the red blood cells make the round trip through the body and back to the heart in about 60 seconds!

Together, your heart and blood vessels make up the *cardiovascular* system, which literally means your *heart* (cardio)-*vessel* (vascular) system. Your blood pressure readings are an important reflection of how well your entire cardiovascular (*heart-vessel*) system is functioning. When your blood pressure is within an optimal range for good health, your blood flows through the vessels of your body without damaging the delicate linings of the vessel walls or creating undue strain on your heart. However, when the heart beats more rapidly (strongly increasing its output of blood), or the arteries are constricted (due to the contraction of the smooth muscles within the vessel walls or by their loss of elasticity), your blood pressure rises. When that happens, your heart has to work harder, pumping blood against greater resistance or higher pressure. That, in turn, increases the stress even further on the heart and arteries.

Simply stated, your blood pressure can rise for three reasons:

1. Your heart beats faster or more strongly, increasing its output of blood (cardiac output).
2. Your arteries constrict, decreasing the overall space through which blood can flow (increased systemic peripheral resistance).
3. A combination of the above.

For a moment, you might imagine the pressure within your vessel walls as similar to water running through a hose. If you increase the volume of water flowing into the hose, the pressure increases. Similarly, if you make the hose narrower, the water presses against the walls of the hose with more force or pressure. Increasing the amount of water flowing into the tubing is like increasing the peripheral resistance in your arteries. A combination of increasing cardiac output and peripheral resistance together only compounds the problem.

Over time, if blood pressure remains high, the situation only becomes worse. The fragile tissues within the vessel walls start to weather and tear. As that happens, another process begins: fat and cholesterol can build up on the vessel walls to compensate for this damage and act as a cushion against the continued turbulence created by the surging blood. These arterial deposits only further impede the blood flow, accelerating damage to the delicate interior of the artery walls. Additional arterial deposits occur, causing the arteries to narrow even more, and the blood pressure to rise still higher.

Thus, a vicious cycle can be set into motion, in which high blood pressure accelerates arteriosclerosis (the narrowing and hardening of the arteries), and arteriosclerosis further raises blood pressure. Fortunately, we now know more about how this degenerative process can be slowed and even reversed; relaxation and stress management techniques and lifestyle modification are the keys to the recovery process.

Under the best and healthiest of conditions, your blood pressure is primarily regulated and fine-tuned by your brain and *Autonomic Nervous System* (ANS). This system controls all the automatic or "involuntary" processes of the body, from the beating of your heart to your blood chemistry. For many people, the ANS functions just fine, making normal adjustments in blood pressure to respond to the varying demands and conditions of everyday life. Throughout the day, the ANS instructs the heart to speed up or slow down, and directs the muscle fibers in the arteries to either constrict the vessels or relax them. When this happens, your blood pressure either rises or falls.

Pressure-sensitive cells called *baroreceptors* play an important role in this system. Contained within the walls of the major arteries—specifically, the aorta and the carotid arteries—the baroreceptors act like thermostats, constantly monitoring and adjusting the arterial blood pressure. The baroreceptors also send messages through electrical impulses that ultimately control arterial constriction and relaxation, as well as alter the activity of the heart.

However, sometimes the system goes awry. If, for instance, there are continuous rises in blood pressure—such as in response to stress—the baroreceptors may increase the level at which they tend to keep your blood pressure. They can start to recognize this higher blood pressure reading as "normal" and maintain it there. This is akin to the thermostat in your home being raised and becoming stuck at a higher setting; the thermostat, like the baroreceptor, is still doing its job, but needs to be reset at a lower level for comfort and health.

This is only a glimpse into some of the components of an intricate, complex, multilevel, and quite remarkable system. When it is in balance and functioning properly, your blood pressure tends to be perfectly controlled. For many people, however, one or more of the components in this system become miscalibrated, whether because of genetic predisposition, response to stress, or poor lifestyle habits.

HYPERTENSION AND THE MIND-BODY CONNECTION

A growing amount of medical research is suggesting the important role of the mind-body connection in controlling hypertension. The evidence now clearly shows that the mind can create changes in the body—and vice versa. In fact, the mind and the body are increasingly being thought of as a unitary system.

If we go back as far as the Hippocratic corpus, medicine of that era recognized that the mind and the body were inseparable. Hippocrates himself said that there is no illness of the body apart from that of the mind. Around the time of Descartes, however, science started to look at the body as a "machine" quite distinct from the mind. The body could be repaired through external agents, scientists argued, leaving no real role for the mind in healing and bringing the body back into balance.

Today, however, medicine is undergoing a transformation toward a more integrated approach; medicine now recognizes that thoughts can influence physiological processes. Through radioimmunoassay technology, for example, scientists have actually been able to observe the chemical changes that occur as an individual reacts in various ways to stress. Chemicals in the brain called neuropeptides have been identified and shown to pass messages to the immune system and the glands, confirming that the body responds to thoughts, images, feelings, and attitudes. Communication is continually occurring along the continuum between mind and body. Some scientists are even now using terms like "the chemistry of thought."

Of course, a multitude of factors, such as genetic predisposition, environment, and lifestyle, are recognized as contributing to the disease process. Increasingly, however, the role of the mind and our responses to stress are being acknowledged as primary influences on who becomes ill or stays well.

THE LINK BETWEEN STRESS AND DISEASE

Dr. Hans Selye, the father of stress research and one of the foremost authorities in the field, defines stress as "the nonspecific response of the body to any demand made upon it." In more common terminology, he describes it as "the rate of wear and tear on the body." Selye found that as people cope with stress in their day-to-day lives, there can be a profound disruption of their equilibrium, both physical and psychological. Selye and other supporters of a stress-disease relationship argue that stressors are capable of making us sick. This theory met with initial skepticism, but as the body of evidence grew, the stress-disease connection eventually became recognized as a factor that could undermine health and well-being.

Many experts, as well as standard medical texts, consider stress to be an important factor in 50 to 80 percent of all illnesses. Stress has been implicated in hypertension, coronary heart disease, cancer, asthma, ulcers, arthritis, low-back pain, alcoholism, headaches, anxiety, depression, impotence, obesity, occupational accidents, suicide, and a host of other problems. Cardiologist Robert Eliot, director of the Institute of Stress Medicine in Denver and a leading authority on the relationship between stress and cardiovascular disease, wrote that "stress may be the greatest single contributor to illness in the industrialized world."

Research by psychiatrist Thomas Holmes and his associate Richard Rahe studied and ranked stressful life changes that appear to make an individual more susceptible to illness. The effect of each stressor was determined by the magnitude of adaptation it required. Minor stressors such as getting a parking ticket required little adaptation, and are near the bottom of this scale of stressful events, whereas the death of a spouse, divorce, and marital separation are stressors with the most severe impact and require the most adjustment. Dr.'s Holmes and Rahe concluded that as stressful events accumulate within a given time period, they increase the chances of disease.

Subsequent research, however, has shown that other influences can mediate or reduce the influence of stress upon our health. Key factors that influence who gets sick and who stays well include our perception or appraisal of the stressor, and whether we feel we are able to cope effectively with it. The power, then, is more within ourselves than in the stress itself.

Drs. David Ornstein and David Sobel have articulated this new understanding in their book *The Healing Brain:*

> The way we perceive and appraise the event, the availability and use of resources to cope with the challenge, have more to do with the outcome than the raw event itself. Stress, and its negative impact on health, derive from a mismatch between perceived environmental demands and perceived resources to adapt.

While some people thrive under stress, others tend to become debilitated and more prone to stress-related disorders. In actuality, there is no way to eliminate all sources of stress in life; however, we can learn skills that break the stress cycle and help prevent the adverse consequences of stress.

Dr. Kenneth Pelletier, director of the Corporate Health Program at the Stanford Center for Research in Disease Prevention, has stated that the individuals who have learned to thrive on stress have incorporated regular islands of peace into their lives, breaking the stress cycle by returning to a relaxed, balanced state of body and mind. Thus, it is not the stress, but how we respond to it that matters. Dr. Selye, in fact, talked about two kinds of stress—*"dis*tress" (which is bad stress) and "eustress" (which is good).

Dr. Elmer and Alyce Green of the Menninger Foundation have pointed out that

> . . . certain types of stress add spice to life. Were it not for stress, sports, as well as much of life, rather than being exhilarating, would be quite dull. According to the Greens, the skier who stands at the top of the mountain who looks down a steep slope and sees both moguls and rocks—and whose blood pressure and heart rate do not increase—probably has something wrong with him. However, if the same skier arrives at the bottom of the mountain and is so terrified by what could have taken place or might happen in the future that his accelerated heart rate and high blood pressure do not go back to normal, then he has the start of a psychosomatic illness. This is an unwanted physical reaction to psychological stress.

THE LINK BETWEEN STRESS AND HIGH BLOOD PRESSURE

To better understand the relationship between stress and hypertension—and how breaking the stress cycle through feedback-assisted deep physiological relaxation and stress management can help reduce your high blood pressure—let's examine some of the physiological and psychological processes that are involved.

The Autonomic Nervous System (ANS) is the part of the nervous system that regulates the body's automatic functions like breathing and the heartbeat. The ANS is divided into two parts—the sympathetic and parasympathetic systems, which counterbalance one another. When stimulated, the sympathetic system accelerates the heart rate and contracts the arteries, whereas the parasympathetic system slows the heart rate and dilates the arteries.

In response to stress or a perceived threat to well-being, the brain—or more specifically, the tiny hypothalamus in the brain that is the mind's central control panel—activates the sympathetic nervous system, which in turn stimulates the body's alarm reaction, commonly referred to as the "fight or flight response." Harvard physiologist Walter Cannon first identified this fight or flight response in the 1920s. Triggering the body's alarm reaction causes a series of rapid, physiological changes, including an escalation of the heart and respiratory rate, an increase in muscle tension, the constriction of blood vessels, a rise in blood pressure, and the release of stress hormones such as *adrenaline* (or *epinephrine*) and *noradrenaline,* which cause the heart to pump even harder. Another hormone, *aldosterone,* is secreted by the adrenal glands, and contributes to the retention of salt and water by the body; when this happens, the blood volume increases, which also leads to higher blood pressure.

Several other substances help regulate—or contribute to the disregulation of—your blood pressure. One of them, an enzyme called *renin,* is secreted by the kidneys and keeps blood pressure from dipping too low. Toward this end, it combines with other chemicals in the bloodstream to produce still other agents, *angiotensin I* and *angiotensin II.* Angiotensin II is a powerful vasoconstrictor, which can create serious problems by constricting or squeezing arterial muscle cells and driving the blood pressure up.

When the instinctive fight or flight response is short-term and in reaction to an immediate threat where fighting or running are appropriate, many of the changes the response stimulates are necessary for survival. For instance, in threatening situations, the acceleration of the heart and breathing rates provides increased blood flow and added oxygen, which supply the extra nutrients and energy our bodies require for either doing battle or running from the source of the threat. The excretion of stress hormones shifts the entire body and mind into high gear; at the same time, the massive constriction of the blood vessels in the arms and legs that the fight or flight response triggers helps retard blood loss that might occur from a wound. Muscular tightening keeps the body's major muscle groups alert and ready for action.

However, if the fight or flight response is triggered frequently and *continuously* by emotional stressors, the effects can become cumulative, resulting in chronic high blood pressure and a breakdown in health. When stressful circumstances are prolonged and our adaptive energy becomes depleted, a host of psychophysiological changes can occur as part of the body's long-term stress response. Under these threatening conditions in which the body tries to support survival over an extended period of time, a "chronic vigilance" reaction is activated, which provokes not only long-term rises in blood pressure, but also impairment of the immune system, the release of fats and cholesterol into the bloodstream, and the retention of sodium by tissues.

Psychologically, this "chronic vigilance" can be accompanied by feelings of being overwhelmed by events or depressed. In contrast to the aggressive stance of the short-term alarm reaction, this response is characterized by withdrawal and decreased interaction with the environment. It is often referred to as *conservation withdrawal.*

Both the short- and long-term responses to stress produce effects opposite to those caused by psychophysiological relaxation, and can contribute to elevations in blood pressure as well as increased wear and tear on the cardiovascular system, including injuries to the lining of the arteries, ruptured heart muscle fibers, and an increased risk of a spasm of the coronary arteries, heart attack, or stroke.

The psychophysiological responses of our early ancestors were more adaptive than they are today. In times when most threats could be dealt with by either physically fighting or fleeing, the exertion of combat or escape burned up stress chemicals and—after the confrontation—the body had a chance to recuperate. Under prolonged states of siege, ongoing vigilance would have contributed to survival; increased fat and cholesterol would have given more staying power in times of famine.

However, the realities of modern life are different. While we have the same trigger-quick psychophysiological programming as our ancestors, it is inappropriate to react to most of today's threatening situations by fighting or fleeing. In our society, most modern "threats" are to our emotional and social well-being; not our immediate physical survival. We are not threatened by charging elephants or saber-toothed tigers, and only rarely encounter a criminal intent on causing harm.

Instead, today's stresses are more likely to be the rising cost of living, highway traffic congestion, discord in personal or work relationships, job insecurity, unemployment, dealing with the needs of children and aging parents, family illness and other social pressures. Rather than being resolved rapidly, these causes of stress—one piled on top of another—can persist for months or even years.

As you have probably surmised, our short-term, highly-reactive physiological responses to stress, as well as our response to long-term stressors, can become part of the problem rather than being helpful. After all, who do you fight when you're caught in intra-office politics or in the middle of bumper-to-bumper traffic? Where do you flee when you're having ongoing financial difficulties or are in the midst of a difficult period of parenting? Faced with repeated and compounded stress, our bodies are on almost constant alert, with little or no time to calm down and regain internal equilibrium, setting us up for stress-related disorders like hypertension.

MORE ABOUT THE STRESS-HYPERTENSION LINK

A number of studies have looked specifically at the relationship between stress and high blood pressure, finding that a strong link does exist. For instance:

> Researchers examined more than 400 air traffic controllers, whose high-pressure jobs require them to remain constantly alert, guiding planes in air-traffic corridors where a single mistake could inadvertently cause hundreds of deaths. Over a three-year period, these controllers developed hypertension at a rate three to four times as high as people of a similar age and sex in the same cities.
>
> When individuals moved from small quiet towns to more stressful urban communities, their blood pressure increased, often to levels within the hypertensive range.

Dr. Eliot has studied individuals who go through life with only occasional escalations of their blood pressure levels. When they are not feeling anxiety, these people may actually have normal blood pressure readings; but even routine stress can result in significant elevations in their blood pressure. Eliot calls these individuals "hot reactors" and has reported that about 17 percent of the U.S. population are physiologically "hyperresponsive" like this. Because these people overtax their cardiovascular systems so excessively, they are prime candidates for heart attacks and other serious health problems.

If your response to stress is part of the problem that contributes to high blood pressure, it makes sense that breaking the stress cycle—through regular deep relaxation and stress management—can be an important part of the solution. As you have read, stress can increase your heart rate, constrict your blood vessels, and raise your blood pressure. Practicing the biobehavioral skills of the HART Program can help bring your body and mind back to a state of equilibrium, evoking a physiological response opposite the fight-or-flight response. Dr. Benson of Harvard Medical School has called this the "relaxation response." By practicing the HART Program's self-regulatory skills, you will slow your heart rate and expand (or vasodilate) your arteries, which will reduce pressure within your blood vessels. As muscles relax, and as the heart rate slows and hands and feet warm, you will quiet the overactivity of your sympathetic nervous system, and your blood pressure will decrease.

FEEDBACK: THE KEY TO SELF-TREATMENT

More than two decades of research and clinical practice in biofeedback and applied psychophysiology demonstrate that we can bring many Autonomic Nervous System (ANS) functions under our control if information about how to do so is made available.

Feedback, of course, is nothing new to human learning. We use it when we learn to drive a car, ride a bike or putt a golf ball into a hole. As we practice and identify what we're doing, figuring out what works and what doesn't, we learn how to improve our skills in these areas. In the same way, obtaining feedback about our internal processes can help us develop the sensitivity and ability to modify our internal physiology in the direction of good health.

Dr. Barbara Brown described this phenomenon in her book *Stress and the Art of Biofeedback:* "When the mind receives information about itself and its body, information about how it reacts to stress and how it can return to well-being, mental faculties of awareness and understanding and control are roused to action. By some obscure capacity, cognitive faculties are set in motion to restore the mind and body to a state of balance and relieve the effects of stress."

In the HART Program, we use a simple mercury thermometer, the type you can purchase in almost any hardware store, to provide an objective indicator of sympathetic nervous system activity.

One of the basic principles of self-regulation is simple: If you can detect what is going on inside your body, you can learn to voluntarily change it in the direction you choose. Different parts of the brain play a role in this learning process. The cortex, along with the voluntary muscular system, influences those bodily functions that we normally consider within our conscious control. The subcortical network, along with the ANS, affect those processes normally outside our conscious awareness.

The limbic system—a specialized area within the subcortical brain—is important in gaining control over these "involuntary" functions. It is often referred to as the visceral or emotional brain, and is extremely responsive to perception and imagination. As we observe external events, stressful or otherwise, our mental and emotional reactions produce a limbic response. In turn, this limbic response activates the hypothalamus, which regulates much of the mechanism of our ANS.

Fortunately, we don't need to fully understand all the mechanisms at work in autonomic regulation—just like you don't need to be aware of the muscles and neural pathways that play a role when you learn to drive a car or ride a bike. Where self-regulation is concerned, the key is to find some external signal—like temperature feedback—that can give the conscious mind information about internal physiological responses. With this new information—and with the help of the HART Program's self-regulatory techniques such as autogenic phrases, Three-Part Complete Breathing, muscular relaxation, and imagery—the mind can learn a new mental and emotional response that eventually results in modifications of the limbic system and hypothalamus. With practice, we can establish voluntary control of normally unconscious processes. When that happens, according to Dr.'s Elmer and Alyce Green, we bridge the gap between the conscious and the unconscious.

Feedback-Assisted Relaxation

In 1974, a medical writer visited the laboratory of the Greens at the Menninger Foundation. The writer was researching an article on the medical applications of biofeedback, and the Greens guided her through a 30-minute exercise in which she progressively relaxed her body from head to toe. In the process, a portable temperature machine showed that her hand temperature had become warmer.

The reporter took the portable machine home with her, and when she returned it a week later, she told the Greens, "You may be interested to know that I got rid of my hypertension last week."

According to the writer, her blood pressure had been 150/90. However, when she had visited her physician at the end of the week—after diligently practicing the relaxation and hand-warming technique—her high blood pressure had decreased to a normal level.

This unexpected and fortuitous discovery became a turning point and springboard for years of research into the role that feedback-assisted relaxation can play in raising peripheral body temperature and, in turn, reducing blood pressure.

Prior to the Greens' discovery, there had been a decade of research utilizing feedback with mostly unsuccessful results. Most of these early studies attempted to use direct blood-pressure feedback—that is, showing a patient moment-by-moment changes in blood pressure, in hopes that an individual could use this information to try to decrease blood pressure. However, this did not prove to be effective. Significant results were achieved only when feedback was used to indicate decreases in sympathetic nervous system activity.

The notable exception among the early researchers was Dr. Chandra Patel and her colleagues from the United Kingdom, who achieved significant success in helping patients lower blood pressure. They first published their findings in the 1970s, describing a successful treatment program consisting of deep relaxation and meditation, assisted by galvanic skin response feedback (which, like temperature feedback, is an indicator of sympathetic nervous system activity), along with training in stress management. Dr. Patel's work, as well as that at the Menninger Voluntary Controls program, continues to be among the most clinically successful in the field.

The first Menninger study by the Greens and Patricia Norris was reported in 1980, and involved a total of nine hypertensive patients in a biobehavioral program. All six patients on antihypertensive medication successfully eliminated their use of these drugs while maintaining their blood pressure at normal levels. One of the patients *not* on antihypertensive medication also achieved a significant decrease in blood pressure (from 139/86 to 111/83) using the relaxation technique.

I have conducted my own review of the clinically successful studies using a biobehavioral approach for the treatment of high blood pressure. An important part of that review was to identify the components within each treatment approach that contributed to reductions in blood pressure and medications. The greatest success was achieved through programs combining biofeedback-assisted relaxation training (where feedback provided an indicator of decreasing sympathetic nervous system activity) with regular home relaxation practice, and in many cases, home monitoring of blood pressure. Stress management was also a significant part of the successful programs, helping patients to transfer their skills to their daily lives.

The following studies illustrate the importance of biofeedback in the successful biobehavioral treatment of high blood pressure:

A controlled study reported by Dr. Keith Sedlacek divided hypertensive patients into two groups. One group learned relaxation techniques accompanied by a biofeedback method; the other used only meditation. After 20 sessions, blood pressure had decreased in the biofeedback-assisted relaxation group from an average of 144/95 to 130/83. These decreases were still evident at a four-month followup evaluation. In addition, 70 percent of the biofeedback patients had their medication cut by 50 percent. By contrast, the meditation-only group showed no significant declines in blood pressure over the four-month period, and thus, they were unable to reduce their medication.

In a study by Dr. Edward Blanchard, 40 hypertensive patients were divided into two groups. Although both groups learned a relaxation technique, only one was also taught thermal feedback and this latter group experienced greater improvements in blood pressure. At the same time, while 13 of 20 patients in the feedback group eliminated one of their antihypertensive medications, only 1 of 20 in the relaxation-only group was able to do so.

Dr. M. Hartfield achieved similar results. Twenty hypertensive patients practiced relaxation training, but only half of them also learned temperature biofeedback for warming hands and feet. In the biofeedback group, systolic and diastolic readings declined 20.6 and 15.4 mm Hg, respectively. By comparison, the nonbiofeedback patients experienced systolic and diastolic decreases of 5.1 and 4.2 mm Hg, respectively. The researchers concluded that temperature biofeedback was an essential component of effective blood pressure reduction.

In this chapter, we have examined the relationship between stress and high blood pressure, and the way in which biobehavioral treatment can help break the stress response. Interestingly, many antihypertensive medications work by creating similar physiological changes to the self-regulatory skills you will learn in this book: they deactivate the overactivity of the sympathetic branch of the nervous system, decrease the heart rate, or increase vasodilation of the arteries. With the HART Program, you can produce the same changes without medications and without side effects.

The next chapter examines the drugs that millions of patients have relied on to control their hypertension.

CHAPTER · 4

Medications: A Change of Heart

*When I came into the HART Program, I was on multiple
medications and my blood pressure was not controlled. Now it
is. My motivation was to reduce blood pressure and dispense
with medication.*

> —HELEN
> Social worker
> HART participant

*I had been taking medication. It wasn't the experience of side
effects that got me interested in the HART program; it was
concern for what the long-range effects might be.*

> —ROBERT
> Attorney
> HART participant

*I've always felt the less medication you take, the better. It just
seems to me I'd be better off if I could lessen my dependence
on medication.*

> —FRANK
> Real estate broker
> HART participant

ALTHOUGH THE HART PROGRAM emphasizes a nondrug biobehavioral
approach to normalizing hypertension, the majority of individuals who
begin the program are on medications when they start. Antihypertensive medications have an important place in the treatment arsenal for
high blood pressure; it is much better to have your blood pressure
under control with drugs than not controlled at all.

Medications can reduce blood pressure, take the strain off the heart
and arteries and help prevent or reduce organ damage and the risk of
cardiovascular disease. However, antihypertensive drugs are not only
costly, they often have unpleasant side effects as well, and the advan-

29

tages drugs provide can also be achieved through nondrug methods of normalizing your blood pressure. A major benefit of the HART Program is that it encourages you to maintain your blood pressure under medically-accepted control as your medications are reduced and hopefully eliminated.

When antihypertensive drugs were first introduced, they were heralded as the cure for high blood pressure. Over the years, they have saved millions of lives. Until these drugs became available, many cases of hypertension were never effectively controlled, sometimes with dire consequences for the affected patients.

However, as beneficial as today's medications can be (and as easy as they are to take) they are unfortunately far from the "miracle cure" for high blood pressure they were first thought to be. Medications may effectively manage the **symptom** of high blood pressure for many patients, yet they do not reverse the **underlying factors** that contribute to this disease. If medications are your only form of treatment to control

---

WHAT KIND OF MEDICATION ARE YOU TAKING?

There are several broad categories of antihypertensive drugs that are commonly prescribed, including the following:

Diuretics cut down the volume of blood and fluids that circulate through the blood vessels by promoting the excretion of sodium and excess water from the body. As this occurs, the pressure on the blood vessels is reduced.

Vasodilators reduce blood pressure by widening the blood vessels. This process occurs as the smooth muscle cells in the arteries relax, resulting in a reduction of resistance within the small arteries. As this resistance declines, so does blood pressure.

Beta-blockers slow down the heart rate, thus cutting back on the pumping activity and the blood output of the heart, which in turn reduces blood pressure.

Calcium-channel blockers are a relatively new type of drug whose mechanism is not well understood. They seem to influence the activity of certain chemicals in the body, which in turn opens up the arteries.

Sympatholytics influence the nervous system's control over the blood vessels, resulting in the dilation of the vessels and a decline in blood pressure.

ACE inhibitors interfere with the activity of an enzyme (the angiotensin converting enzyme) that appears to play an important role in the development of hypertension in many patients.

your blood pressure, you will most likely need to take them for the rest of your life.

Until fairly recently, hypertension was thought to be an incurable disorder requiring life-long medication management. Fortunately, from what we now know about nonpharmacological methods for blood pressure control, this is no longer considered to be the case.

"STEPPED CARE" NOW INCLUDES "STEP ZERO"

The Joint National Committee on Detection, Evaluation, and Treatment of High Blood Pressure has recommended that physicians used a "stepped care" approach for prescribing medication. Under this procedure, the patient starts at a small dosage of one drug, and if necessary, the dosage is gradually increased. Then, other drugs are added or substituted, and dosages are gradually raised until blood pressure is brought under control.

For the first time, however, an approach called "step zero" is also now being recommended. With the "step zero" procedure, medication is gradually reduced and then eliminated for individuals who can regain control of their blood pressure through nonpharmacological means.

That is good news, and for a number of reasons. Antihypertension drugs can cost, on average, from $400 to $1,000 a year. Over a few decades, this adds up to a considerable sum. Escalating insurance rates and Medicare and Medicaid costs indicate that someone is bearing this expense.

Cost, however, is usually not the primary concern. Even more troubling, all medications have potential side effects, which can detract from quality of life and in some cases even contribute to longer-term health problems. At least 22 adverse effects of antihypertensive drugs have been reported, ranging from chronic fatigue to depression. Sex-related side effects, including impotence and retrograde ejaculation, are widely recognized in males. Most people, however, are unaware that antihypertensive medications can also decrease sexual interest, as well as vaginal lubrication, in women.

Some long-term side effects may also increase the risk of cardiovascular disease. Studies have documented, for example, that extended use of beta-blockers can contribute to increases in atherosclerosis and triglycerides, and decreases in protective HDL (High-Density Lipoprotein) cholesterol. A large-scale clinical trial found that diuretics can be associated with an increased risk of early death in patients whose electrocardiograms show signs of abnormal functioning.

Not everyone experiences adverse effects from these drugs. However, a study by Drs. William Stason and Milton Weinstein of the Harvard School of Public Health showed that the average patient has from two to four side effects, any of which can undermine his or her quality of life. And for individuals taking multiple antihypertensive medications, interactions among these drugs may only further increase these difficulties.

Some patients just accept side effects as the price they have to pay for the control of their hypertension. At least they feel that way in the beginning. Yet many eventually tire of these adverse effects and stop taking their medication, leaving their blood pressure uncontrolled and their health at risk. According to the National Heart, Lung, and Blood Institute, after five years, 80 percent of patients no longer follow their prescribed course of medication.

As a result, the American Medical Association has concluded that **only approximately one in seven Americans with hypertension receives adequate treatment.**

This distressing statistic as well as the other problems attendant to the management of hypertension by medication contributed to the recent change of policy regarding how best to treat high blood pressure. Most individuals who now choose biobehavioral treatment and lifestyle modification do so specifically because they are viable alternatives to the long-term use of medication. Many HART patients have stated that they are uncomfortable with the idea that they must rely on a pill for something as important as their blood pressure. Others are concerned about possible long-term side effects and want to get off medications for that reason.

ADVERSE EFFECTS ASSOCIATED WITH THE MOST COMMONLY-PRESCRIBED HYPERTENSIVE DRUGS ——————

Diuretics	hypokalemia (blood potassium deficiency), hyperkalemia (excessive blood potassium), hyperuricemia (excessive uric acid in the blood), glucose intolerance, high blood cholesterol level, high blood triglyceride level, sexual dysfunction, male breast development, breast pain
Beta-blockers	bradycardia (slow heart beat), fatigue, insomnia, bizarre dreams, sexual dysfunction, low HDL cholesterol level, high blood triglyceride level

Calcium-channel blockers	headache, excessively low blood pressure, nausea, flushing, constipation, edema
Vasodilators	headache, tachycardia (abnormally fast heart beat), fluid retention, excessive hair growth
Sympatholytics	drowsiness, dry mouth, fatigue, sexual dysfunction
ACE inhibitors	rash, impaired sense of taste

Not only are there no known adverse side effects from biobehavioral treatment, but patients report many positive effects in their lives, from feeling more in control of stress and better about themselves to improved relationships with other people. More importantly, biobehavioral treatment goes beyond symptomatic control of blood pressure. The techniques you will learn in this program can actually address and remedy some of the underlying problems contributing to your high blood pressure.

Reducing and eliminating medication may be a priority for you. However, it is important that **if you are presently taking medication for your high blood pressure, you continue to do so as you start this program and that you only make medication changes with the support and supervision of your physician.** As you regain control of your blood pressure through your practice of self-regulatory techniques and other lifestyle modifications, your doctor will help you determine when gradual reductions in medication are in order. **Only your physician should recommend and supervise any medication adjustments.** Drugs can keep your hypertension under control while you are learning HART's nondrug approach to reducing your blood pressure. **Lowering your medication on your own, or changing your dosage too abruptly, could be hazardous to your health.**

GUIDELINES FOR REDUCING AND ELIMINATING MEDICATIONS

If you are currently taking medication to control your blood pressure, follow your prescribed medication regimen, making adjustments only with your doctor's approval. These guidelines for adjusting medication dosages are based on those that have been in clinical use at the Menninger Foundation's Voluntary Control program:

1. Once you have established a regular system of relaxation practice and recordkeeping, keep your doctor apprised of your progress. Contact your physician about the possibility of reducing your medication each time you manage to keep your average pre-relaxation blood pressure at 140/90 mm Hg or less over a two-week period. Do this until all medications are eliminated. In this way, you will slowly taper off the medication while keeping your blood pressure under medically-acceptable control. Your own blood pressure records can assist your physician in making an informed decision.

2. All changes in your use of prescribed medications must be made only through consultation with your physician—never on your own. Also, these changes need to be gradual; do not abruptly discontinue medication, as this could be hazardous to your health.

3. In most cases, centrally-active (such as Catapres) and peripherally-active medications (such as Serpasil) are gradually reduced first until they are completely discontinued. Next, your doctor may gradually reduce and eliminate diuretics.

4. By practicing self-regulatory techniques and health-oriented lifestyle changes, you may also reduce your need for medications taken for other medical conditions—for example, the insulin requirements for an individual with diabetes may decrease. Inform your physician of *all* medications you may be taking. Let your doctor know you are participating in a program that may require reducing medications other than those you are taking for your blood pressure.

HOW TO WORK WITH YOUR DOCTOR

The majority of my patients find their doctor understanding and supportive of their preference to use nondrug methods to control their blood pressure. If your objective is to normalize your blood pressure through biobehavioral and/or other nonpharmacological methods, it is important to familiarize yourself with the protocol for making medication reductions, and then discuss the program with your doctor. Consult your physician about setting reasonable blood pressure goals, and ask for his or her support.

Let your physician know you will be keeping daily blood pressure records and that you will want to confer with him whenever your blood pressure stabilizes at or below 140/90 for a two-week period to see if a medication adjustment is appropriate. Because the HART techniques

will very likely reduce your blood pressure, your medication will require periodic adjustments so you will not be overmedicated and become hypotensive (blood pressure below normal). Please do not stop or
decrease your medication without your doctor's supervision.

Patients and their doctors can decide if the HART Program works by
looking at its results. Nothing speaks louder than your blood pressure
records. If your blood pressure readings decline and stay within
medically-acceptable limits as you **gradually** taper off and finally eliminate medications, you will know that the program is working for you.
It is important to be patient; your high blood pressure took time to
develop, and you will need time to normalize it.

On rare occasions, patients find their doctor uninterested in reducing
their medication, even if their blood pressure has stabilized well within
the low-normal range. If you find yourself in this situation, discuss your
goals and concerns with your physician. You may consider suggesting a
small reduction for a trial period and monitoring the results both with
home and office measurements.

Some doctors are more oriented toward taking a biobehavioral and
lifestyle approach to blood pressure control. Physician Herbert Benson
of Boston's Beth Israel Hospital makes these recommendations for
choosing your doctor:

> Find a supportive doctor whom you trust. . . You can never overestimate
> the importance of warmth, concern and a trust-inspiring style on the part
> of the physician. . . So I would strongly recommend that you be aggressive
> (assertive) . . . in picking the doctor who is right for you and 'on your wave
> length.' Don't assume that every doctor is the same . . . [I]f the first phy-
> sician you contact doesn't seem quite right . . . find the one whose style and
> manner are consistent with and supportive of your own.

Working with a doctor supportive of your goals is immensely helpful,
and may have major consequences for your health.

CHAPTER 5

Blood Pressure, Risk & Longevity: Why Lower Your Blood Pressure?

A lower level of blood pressure will, in fact, lower the risk for the complications of stroke and coronary artery heart disease. The risk rate, however, begins to rise very substantially when the systolic pressure begins to exceed 140 or the diastolic pressure begins to exceed 90.

—Dr. Edward Lichter, M.D.
University of Illinois

Nonpharmacologic intervention . . . needs to be a part of the antihypertensive treatment of all patients.

—Rose Stamler, M.A.
Jeremiah Stamler, M.D.
Northwestern University
Medical School

If you have hypertension, your doctor has probably discussed the need for you to bring your blood pressure down. He or she may have recommended that you relax more, reduce the salt and cholesterol in your diet, and increase your exercise.

A major reason for the increased attention to managing hypertension without the use of drugs is the recent redefinition of high blood pressure. In its 1984 report, the Joint National Committee on Detection, Evaluation, and Treatment of High Blood Pressure—a policymaking panel composed of the nation's leading experts on hypertension—lowered the threshold of high blood pressure from 160/95 to 140/90 mm Hg. In other words, a blood pressure of 160/95 mm Hg is no longer considered the point at which high blood pressure is diagnosed; persons with an even lower blood pressure—specifically, 140/90 mm Hg—are now classified as hypertensive.

When the joint national committee announced this major change in the definition of high blood pressure, 40 million more Americans automatically found themselves in the "at risk" category. No longer, for example, will individuals with 140/90 be told by their doctor that their blood pressure is normal. Rather than being considered "healthy," they are now candidates for some type of treatment.

Under the new reclassification, nearly one in three Americans is considered to have hypertension. And unfortunately, many of these people with high blood pressure are undiagnosed and therefore go untreated. According to the the new committee report, the number of hypertensives aware of their disorder has declined from 74 to 59 percent, the percentage of those taking antihypertensive drugs has fallen from 56 to 33 percent, and the number of hypertensives who have their hypertension under control has decreased from 34 to 11 percent.

CLASSIFICATION OF BLOOD PRESSURE IN ADULTS ⸻

Diastolic blood pressure

less than 85	normal
85–89	high normal
90–104	mild hypertension
105–114	moderate hypertension
over 115	severe hypertension

Systolic blood pressure (when dystolic is under 90 mm Hg)

less than 140	normal
140–159	borderline isolated systolic hypertension
over 160	isolated systolic hypertension

For your own health and longevity, it makes sense to take the new joint national committee guidelines seriously. Set a goal to keep your blood pressure under 140/90 or substantially under that level if you can. What is a good pressure for you? This is something that you should discuss with your doctor.

Dr. Norman Kaplan, an acknowledged authority on hypertension and a member of the joint national committee, considers 120/80 a reasonable goal for most people. Actuarial studies have identified 100/65 as the blood pressure associated with the least risk of cardiovascular disease and the longest expected life span.[2] However, there is some concern about using antihypertensive drugs to keep blood pressure **too**

How Many Hypertensives Fall Into Each Blood Pressure Category? What Percentage Are On Medication?

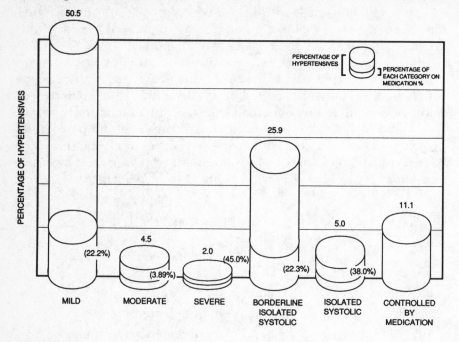

NOTE: Hypertension is defined as 140/90 mmHg or above or currently taking antihypertensive medication.

SOURCE: NHANES II

low because it may be associated with an increased risk of heart attacks; this higher risk, however, has **not** been linked with the biobehavioral approach which normalizes your blood pressure.

WHO IS SUSCEPTIBLE TO HIGH BLOOD PRESSURE?

Do you have a family history of hypertension? Heredity is a primary factor influencing susceptibility to high blood pressure. If one of your parents had hypertension, there is a 50 percent chance that you will develop high blood pressure. If both parents had hypertension, the likelihood increases to 90 percent.

Hypertension is a progressive disorder. If you have "high-normal" readings at an early age, your blood pressure may go up even more over time. The blood pressure in many people inches up as they get older until it is officially diagnosed as being high, sometimes as early as their thirties or forties. For that reason, the earlier you take steps to keep your blood pressure down, the better.

In some people, blood vessels become less elastic and pliable with age, and this rigidity contributes to a rise in systolic blood pressure. About 65 percent of individuals age 65 to 74 have hypertension as a result.

In some cultures, however, older people do not tend to have high blood pressure more frequently than younger ones. Thus, it is not a biological given that blood pressure absolutely increases with age: this elevation may instead be largely related to lifestyle typical of many in Western and industrialized countries, which includes poor eating and exercise habits, and high stress levels.

Although more younger men than women have high blood pressure, women who are pregnant or taking birth control pills are more susceptible to developing essential hypertension. Women become much more vulnerable after menopause, too. The hypertension rate for females age 55 to 64 is actually equal to that of males in the same age group, and then even exceeds the rate for men in the following decade of life.

There is also a somewhat higher incidence of hypertension in Afro-American men (38 percent) as compared to Caucasian men (33 percent). In females, however, the differences are much more striking: Afro-American women have a 69 percent higher incidence of hypertension than Caucasian women.

But no matter what your age, sex, or race, as your blood pressure rises, so do your health risks. As Dr. Norman Kaplan has written, "The higher the blood pressure, the greater the morbidity and mortality."

Just how grave are the statistics? About 31,000 Americans die each year because of high blood pressure. Those are a lot of lives lost. Even so, this is a deceptively low statistic when you consider that of the approximately 2 million deaths in the U.S. each year, almost half (982,000 in 1988) are due to cardiovascular disease, to which high blood pressure is a major contributing factor. In fact, cardiovascular disease is the number one health problem and the major cause of death in developed nations. WHO, the World Health Organization, is currently engaging in a longitudinal 27-nation study entitled MONICA—MONItoring of trends and determinants in CARdiovascular disease. **Hypertension is one of the leading risk factors for cardiovascular disease (CVD). If your hypertension is uncontrolled, you have an increased chance of suffering a heart attack, a stroke, congestive heart failure, coronary heart disease, and kidney disease—even if your blood pressure indicates only mild to moderate hypertension.** In fact, authorities in the field of hypertension such as Dr. Kaplan and Drs. Jeremiah and Rose Stamler believe that the term "mild hypertension" is a misnomer because the people classified as "mild" account for most of the illness, disability, and death attributed to high blood pressure each year.

THE CARDIOVASCULAR RISKS OF HIGH BLOOD PRESSURE

Hypertension is an underlying risk factor for atherosclerosis, heart attacks, strokes, and eye and kidney disease. All are intimately interconnected, and in a number of ways. The clogged and obstructed blood vessels characteristic of atherosclerosis force your heart to work harder; at the same time, there is a rise in the overall pressure of the blood against the artery walls, reflected in higher blood pressure readings.

As your blood pressure increases, so does your risk of a heart attack or a stroke. A *heart attack* (also called a *myocardial infarction*) takes place when the blood flow to the heart is severely impeded or blocked. If this obstruction continues, the heart muscle will receive insufficient nourishment; when the heart is cut off from oxygen and the blood supply, the individual is at serious risk for premature death.

A *stroke* occurs when a blood vessel that supplies oxygen to the brain ruptures or is blocked by a blood clot (thrombus), thus depriving brain cells of oxygen and causing brain damage, disability, or even death. The vessels that the brain depends on are the carotid arteries, located on either side of the throat, and the vertebral arteries that travel up the back of the neck. High blood pressure over a lengthy period can increase the chances of a stroke, due to the constant stress and subsequent weakening of these artery walls, which eventually results in a cerebral or brain hemorrhage.

Many other organs of the body bear the brunt of this disease process. As atherosclerosis narrows the vessels that nourish the eyes with blood and oxygen, damage to the retina and visual problems can occur. As atherosclerosis worsens, the thickening renal (or kidney) vessels become less efficient at supplying the kidneys with blood. This can interfere with normal kidney functioning, including controlling the flow of urine and the filtering of toxins out of the blood and the body. Even though there may be no obvious symptoms, individuals may start to retain large amounts of fluid. With this increased stress upon the kidneys, blood pressure can rise even higher. Ultimately, the kidneys can take only so much, and with the increased wear and tear, renal failure can occur, forcing the need for kidney transplants or dependence on a dialysis machine.

High blood pressure is an underlying risk factor of these cardiovascular diseases (CVD), which can lead to premature disability and death. Fortunately, the incidence of CVD is on a decline: the number of strokes, for example, has decreased markedly in recent years. Even so, if current trends continue, more than one in four Americans can expect to experience some type of cardiovascular disease during his or her lifetime. Once you begin to consider the scope of CVD—nearly 66 million Americans presently suffer from some type of it—then the dangers of hypertension become much more clear.

CONTROLLING THE RISK FACTORS

If you have hypertension, all evidence indicates that you should not just ignore it and hope it goes away. Your risk of coronary heart disease increases as the number of risk factors goes up. For instance, while hypertension, high blood cholesterol, stress, smoking, obesity, and diabetes can each contribute to heart disease, your risk rises approximately **four-fold** if you have two of these factors. When three factors are present, your risk increases **eight** times.

Stress, which is a major focus of the HART Program, is another important risk factor of CVD. Stress can cause irregular heart beats and chaotic heart rhythms that can actually contribute to sudden cardiac death—a phenomenon that kills about 1,200 people a day in the U.S., or about one death per minute. Sudden cardiac death is responsible for about 60 percent of deaths from coronary artery disease.

Cardiologist Robert Eliot, in *Is It Worth Dying For?*, wrote:

> The major traditional risk factors—high blood pressure, high cholesterol, diabetes, obesity and smoking—fail to explain approximately half of the world-wide cases of coronary heart disease. There is good reason to believe that stress is a major missing piece of the puzzle. Moreover, researchers are increasingly recognizing not only that stress is an independent contributor to heart disease, but also that it is closely interwoven with the five traditional risk factors. *Controlling unnecessary stress may therefore be the single most important key to preventing heart attacks.*

Some of the risk factors that may contribute to CVD—such as heredity, increasing age, and being male—can't be changed. But others—including hypertension, stress, high blood cholesterol, obesity, diabetes, and smoking—can be altered. To improve your chances for good health, it makes sense to manage those risks that are within your control.

The HART Program not only helps you reduce your blood pressure, it will also decrease many of the other CVD risk factors. The biobehavioral aspects of the HART Program help minimize the effects of stress upon your health and enable you to reduce your blood pressure. Eating a diet lower in salt and fat, and higher in complex carbohydrates, protective minerals, and vitamins, and shedding excess pounds also help to lower blood pressure and decrease the risk of cardiovascular disease.

There are substantive reasons, then, for controlling high blood pressure. Normalizing your hypertension helps:

prevent damage to the arteries and vital organs

reduce your risk of "cardiovascular accident"—that is, heart attacks, stroke and congestive heart failure, as well as kidney disease and brain injury

increase your expected life span.

The message is clear: To protect your health and longevity, make normalizing your blood pressure—and reducing other cardiovascular risk factors—a priority in your life.

PART II

The HART Techniques for the Self-Regulation of Blood Pressure

---

CHAPTER 6

Taking Your Blood Pressure for Life

Taking blood pressure is one of the most important parts of the program. I had never realized what blood pressure was and what it meant, because I had never felt it. Taking my blood pressure during the training program made me more aware of how blood pressure fluctuates up and down. Under stressful situations, I could see that my pressure was high. I became aware of it and then took steps to relax.

—STAN
Venture capital executive
HART participant

KNOWLEDGE IS POWER; as you learn what is affecting the "ups and downs" of your blood pressure, you will be better able to make the changes that can help normalize your readings.

In this program, you will be asked to take and record your blood pressure and pulse each day. Regular measurements will provide you with a valuable, high-quality source of information to track your progress in regaining control over your high blood pressure. In addition, if you're taking antihypertensive medication, only regular blood pressure monitoring will tell you when you have gained enough self-regulatory control of your blood pressure for your doctor to taper and eventually eliminate your medication.

Taking and recording your blood pressure and pulse rate once each day, both before and after your relaxation practice will help you determine which relaxation techniques work best for you. By reviewing your records over time, you will increase your insight into how your response to different situations or lifestyle habits may be affecting your blood pressure. For instance, what effect is stress having on your blood pressure? What about the influence of dietary changes? Or exercise?

The **only** way to really know your blood pressure at any given time is to measure it. This chapter guides you through a ten-step technique for doing just that.

If measuring your own blood pressure seems intimidating at this point, don't despair. Even people who are initially hesitant learn this technique quickly and soon start to experience the benefits of self-monitoring. Jerry, a graduate of the program, put it this way: "I like the fact that I can have some control over measuring my blood pressure and understanding what it is really doing, instead of letting the doctor or nurse tell me. With a little bit of training, I think anyone can do it. It's not that complicated."

Once Jerry began to monitor and control his blood pressure, he developed a greater sense of control over his own health and well-being. "I like feeling that I'm not totally dependent on others," he told me. "The medical profession is doing the best it can. But it's still my body, and I like the idea of being able to care for it."

Another patient, Mark, related how anxious he had felt in the month-long interim between doctor's appointments, waiting to find out his blood pressure readings. He reported being immensely relieved at having immediate access to this information once had had learned to take his own pressure. According to Mark, "Monitoring my own blood pressure has been liberating for me. . . Now I can check my blood pressure without a second party being involved. This monitoring has become part of my life."

Not too many years ago, doctors usually discouraged their patients from monitoring and recording their blood pressure at home. This is now changing. Many doctors now prescribe this procedure for patients who are willing and able to do so. In fact, the Joint National Committee on Detection, Evaluation, and Treatment of High Blood Pressure has encouraged the active participation of patients in antihypertensive programs, which include self-monitoring of blood pressure.

Your physician will also be able to make good use of your blood pressure measurement records. Under ordinary circumstances, your doctor probably measures your blood pressure only when you make your quarterly or annual office visit. These occasional measurements can be skewed by the phenomenon known as "white coat hypertension," in which individuals (like Mark) might have higher blood pressure readings in their doctors' offices, perhaps due to anxiety about their blood pressure and health. Being able to provide your doctor with your home records will give him or her much more data to help evaluate how your blood pressure is responding to the HART Program, and what medication adjustments should be made.

ORIGINS OF BLOOD PRESSURE MEASUREMENT

In the early eighteenth century, a man named Stephen Hales took the first blood pressure measurement. He was a Church of England clergyman, who also had an enduring fascination with science. With a crowd gathered around him, he used a brass needle and a vertical glass tube to measure the blood pressure of a horse. Hales inserted the needle into the mare's carotid artery, and the blood shot up to about the nine-foot mark of the thirteen-foot-long tube. Hales took repeated measurements, and as the horse became calmer over time, its blood pressure gradually declined.

The measuring of blood pressure in humans went through several evolutions, as early scientists tried to devise a technique that would not require the puncturing of an artery. Finally, in 1896, Scipione Riva-Rocci, an Italian doctor, came up with the idea of putting an inflatable cuff around the arm, and filling it with air until the pulse at the wrist disappeared. This cuff was connected to a glass tube filled with mercury, which responded to pressure within the artery. Using this technique, he was able to obtain a rough measurement of systolic blood pressure.

HOW BLOOD PRESSURE MEASUREMENT WORKS

Today, measuring blood pressure is simpler yet more sophisticated. In this program, you will use a *sphygmomanometer* (pronounced: sfig' mo ma nom' e ter), a device that allows you to listen to arterial sounds while keeping an eye on a measuring dial. This piece of hardware consists of several components: a compression cuff containing an inflatable bag or "bladder" that wraps around your upper arm; a stethoscope or microphone for picking up the pulsating sounds within your arteries; and a pressure gauge or column of mercury that measures your blood pressure.

As you will soon find out, the sphygmomanometer is harder to pronounce than it is to use. Briefly, here's how its elements work together to provide systolic and diastolic blood pressure measurements. With the cuff wrapped around your arm, you fill it with air until the major artery in your arm (the brachial artery) is squeezed so tightly that you have temporarily occluded or cut off the flow of blood through it. Then, you let a small amount of air out of the cuff, decreasing pressure on the artery. When the pressure in the cuff is equal to the pressure in the artery, the blood begins to push its way along the once-closed artery. At that moment, you will hear the first tapping sound through the stethoscope; this correponds to your *systolic* reading.

Then, as you release more air from the cuff, the artery eventually opens fully, the blood starts to flow without obstruction, and the sound in the artery disappears. The moment the sound disappears corresponds to the *diastolic* reading, which represents the pressure in the arteries when the heart is between beats, filling up with blood.

What the Sounds Mean

The sounds you hear through the stethoscope are called Korotkoff's sounds, which were first described by Russian physiologist Nikolai Korotkoff in 1905. Historically, these noises were attributed solely to changes in the blood flow within the arteries. More recently, however, some researchers have identified complex vibrations within the walls of the arteries that may actually be responsible for these sounds. While the vibrations may originate within the walls themselves or within the blood, they appear unrelated to the rate of blood flow.

KOROTKOFF'S SOUNDS

Researchers have divided Korotkoff's sounds into five phases. For our purposes, phases 1 and 5 are the most important.

Phase 1   The first appearance of clear, tapping sounds that gradually increase in intensity. This represents the systolic blood pressure.

Phase 2   The sounds change to a murmur and have a swishing quality. This occurs while the blood is flowing from the constricted artery into the wider artery. (Sometimes, all sound briefly disappears between the tapping of phase 1 and the onset of phase 3, a period known as an *ausculatory gap*.)

Phase 3   The sounds take on a loud, knocking quality, but are not quite as clear as those in phase 1. This occurs when the cuff pressure is further decreased. As that happens, the arteries open when the heart contracts, then close as the heart relaxes.

Phase 4   The sounds become muffled suddenly and again have a faint, swishing quality. This occurs when the pressure in the cuff becomes lower than the arterial pressure. The artery remains open during both the contractions and expansions of the heart.

Phase 5   All sounds disappear.

CHOOSING YOUR BLOOD PRESSURE MEASUREMENT DEVICE

When shopping for a sphygmomanometer, you will find three types to choose from: aneroid models, electronic models, and mercury column models.

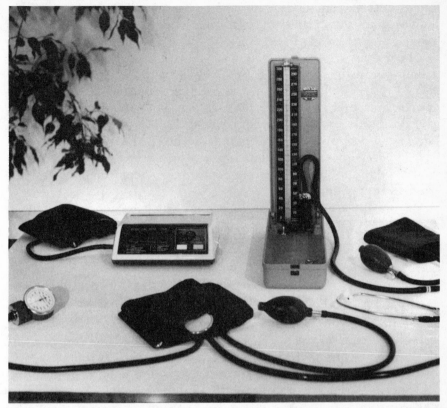

The three types of blood pressure measuring devices: *foreground,* an aneroid model with the stethoscope head built into the cuff; *left,* an electronic model; *right,* a mercury column device.

Although you can use any of these devices in the program, your best choice is an aneroid unit specifically designed for home self-measurement, with the stethoscope head built directly into the cuff. The aneroid unit has a round, clock-like gauge with a needle that points to the increments on the dial face that you will read to determine your blood pressure. This model is considerably easier and less cumbersome to use than a regular aneroid or mercury column unit, both of which have separate stethoscopes. (Many HART patients who purchased a device with a built-in stethoscope—even though they already owned another model—were happy they did.)

Electronic sphygmomanometers have increased in popularity in recent years. They are easy to use and usually provide a "digital" readout of your blood pressure measurement. If your hearing or vision is impaired, or you have problems with manual dexterity that could interfere with your use of an aneroid self-measurement unit, then an electronic model is probably your best choice. However, while the aneroid units have tended to provide greater accuracy in detecting the subtler sounds associated with your diastolic pressure, some electronic models are increasing in accuracy.

The mercury column models, which have a long glass tube filled with mercury, are the kind you'll probably see in your doctor's office attached to the wall. Although they are the most accurate and reliable instruments, they are bulkier, more fragile, and more difficult to use. If you do decide to use a mercury model, keep it away from children, since if it is dropped, the toxic mercury could escape from the reservoir.

No matter what type of unit you eventually select, you will probably find it sold as a kit in places like pharmacies, department stores, and medical supply houses.

State-of-the-art blood pressure equipment is changing rapidly. If you would like recommendations for selecting monitoring equipment currently available, send a self-addressed, stamped envelope to the HART Institute, 645 N. Michigan Ave., Suite 800, Chicago, IL 60611.

CHOOSING THE RIGHT SIZE CUFF

When making your selection of blood pressure measurement devices, be sure to choose a properly-fitted cuff. Most home blood pressure devices come equipped with *standard* adult-size cuffs. If you are a large or very muscular person (whose arm at its widest point measures thirteen inches (33 cm) or more) you will need to purchase a *large* adult size cuff in order to obtain accurate blood pressure readings. If the cuff is too small, you may get falsely elevated readings. One study found that as many as 37 percent of very overweight individuals were falsely diagnosed as having hypertension because a large adult cuff was not used. If you are taking a child's blood pressure, shop for a small, child-sized cuff.

The instructions below for measuring your blood pressure are for use with an aneroid self-measurement model, with either a built-in or a separate stethoscope. Even so, the basics of blood pressure measurement are similar, no matter what type of unit you have. You will need to modify your technique, however, if you are using other kinds of equipment (review the printed manufacturer's instructions provided with your unit).

TAKING YOUR BLOOD PRESSURE

Measuring your own blood pressure is easier than you might think. Like learning any new skill, it will take some time and practice to master the technique. Yet even patients who do not consider themselves mechanically inclined become quite proficient very rapidly. You might feel a bit awkward at first, as if you are working with an octopus and it might be easier if you had a few more arms yourself. This is another reason to purchase a device with a built-in stethoscope head, because it will not require the third arm you don't have. In the beginning, you'll probably have to practice putting the cuff on your arm, adjusting the value on the gauge, and identifying the tapping sounds you'll hear through the stethoscope a few times before you feel at ease. But after a while, the technique will become second nature.

Claire is a concert pianist, the mother of four, and the grandmother of two. When she first began the HART Program, she was hesitant to take her blood pressure, because it looked as though it might be too complicated or too time-consuming.

However, with encouragement, Claire gave it a try. Near the end of her first self-monitoring session—with the cuff on her arm and the gauge in her hand—she looked up with twinkling eyes and said, "This is fun!" Claire now has the satisfaction and sense of accomplishment and control that taking her own blood pressure brings. She now checks her blood pressure before and after each relaxation session and feels good about her blood pressure readings, which have been decreasing steadily since she began the program.

In the beginning, take your time. Allow yourself 30 to 45 minutes to go through the ten steps, moving methodically from one to the next. **Every** step is important. If a particular stage turns out to be especially challenging for you, practice it a few times before moving on. Once you have learned to do it correctly, then you will be measuring your *actual* blood pressure each time, rather than *changes* in the way you measure it. Measuring your blood pressure will really take less than an hour to learn. Once you are at ease with taking your blood pressure, it will take you only a few minutes each time, and it's a skill you can use for life.

To get started, use a chair with a back that will support your own back as you take your blood pressure. You will also need a high table or desk—not only to support your arm with the cuff at heart height, but also as a place to put your blood pressure measuring device, a watch or clock with a second hand or digital display for taking your pulse, a pen or pencil, paper, and your Daily Blood Pressure log (found on page 57). Both your vision and hearing need to be acute in order to take an accurate measurement; if you use glasses or a hearing aid, make sure they're handy, too.

Also, taking your blood pressure is easier if you wear a sleeveless or short-sleeved garment. If you are wearing long sleeves and need to roll them up to bare your upper arm, make sure the shirt or blouse is not so tight that it constricts your blood flow. If you can place two fingers under your sleeve, the garment fits just fine.

Place your equipment and materials within reach on the table, and take a few minutes to familiarize yourself with the blood pressure gauge. The dial of the gauge, like the face of a clock, has both short and long lines around its circumference: each shorter line represents two millimeters of mercury, while each longer line represents ten millimeters of mercury.

When taking your blood pressure, cultivating a relaxed, objective frame of mind not only helps ensure an accurate reading, it is a lot kinder to your nervous system. If your blood pressure ever turns out to be higher than you expected, take a few deep breaths, relax, and take another reading.

It's time to get started.

TEN STEPS TO TAKING YOUR BLOOD PRESSURE

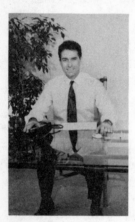

Sit quietly

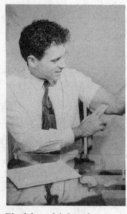

Find brachial pulse

1. Sit quietly for a few minutes before taking your blood pressure. It is best to be in a quiet place, free of distractions, since you'll need to listen carefully for tapping sounds through the stethoscope.
2. Sit with your arm extended and your palm up, slightly bent, and resting comfortably on a table at about the same level as your heart. Your back should be supported by your chair. Keep your legs uncrossed and rest your feet flat on the floor. (If you assume other positions, such as sitting with your back unsupported, standing, or reclining, your measurements will probably be different than those you get while seated with your back supported.) Then bare the skin of your upper, nondominant arm, making sure that if you are wearing long sleeves, your rolled sleeve is not constricting blood flow. You should be able to place at least two fingers under your sleeve.
3. The sounds that help you determine your blood pressure come from your brachial pulse. To find it, bend your arm at the elbow, positioning your forearm at a right angle. Make a fist so your upper arm muscles bulge. Just above the center of the upper arm, you will see or feel (by gentle probing) an indentation whereyour bicep and tricep

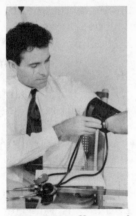

Wrap the cuff around your arm

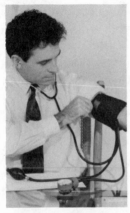

Position cuff, stethoscope, and gauge

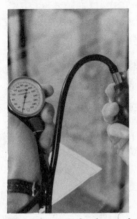

Close the metal valve and inflate the cuff

muscles meet. With a gentle but firm touch, using the pads of your middle and forefingers, press into that space or indentation in the belly of the muscle until you feel a pulsing. This is your brachial artery pulse. Remember where it is located since you will be positioning the head of your stethoscope over this point.

4. Make sure the rubber tubing is coming out of the bottom of the cuff. Wrap the cuff snugly around your upper arm so the lower edge of the cuff is just above the bend of your elbow. The cuff should be smooth, unwrinkled, and wrapped around your skin, not your clothing. If you are using a cuff with a built-in stethoscope, **the head of the stethoscope should be positioned on top of your brachial artery pulse.** If you are using a blood pressure unit with a separate stethoscope, position the cuff so it is one inch above your elbow crease.

Place the head of the stethoscope over your brachial artery pulse firmly but lightly, so its full circumference is in contact with the skin. Keep the stethoscope head from rubbing against tubing or clothing to prevent extraneous noise.

Adjust the pliable metal ear pieces of the stethoscope to your head size for comfort. Place the stethoscope ear pieces in your ears, with the plastic tips angled forward.

For the next step, either hold the round gauge so you can see the dial, or, if you prefer your hands free, clip the gauge onto its box or some other support. Make sure you can look straight at the dial so you will read it more accurately.

5. Close the metal valve just below the rubber bulb by turning the valve clockwise. Don't tighten the valve so much that you have to wrestle it open, but do close it completely. Then inflate the cuff by rapidly squeezing the rubber bulb. You will be able to feel the cuff tightening. Watch the hand on the dial

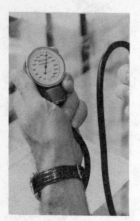

Deflate the cuff

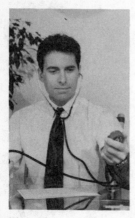

Listen for sounds

of the gauge as you continue increasing the pressure in the cuff. Inflate the cuff until the gauge reads approximately 30 mm Hg above your systolic pressure. For example, if your systolic pressure is usually 170 mm Hg, raise the dial reading to 200. If you are uncertain what your systolic pressure usually is, inflate the cuff to 210.

6. Open the metal valve a little bit by turning it very slightly counterclockwise. Gradually and smoothly, adjust the valve as needed to deflate the cuff at the slow, steady rate of 2 to 3 mm Hg per second. This means you want to see the hand on the dial pulse two to three times within the two longer lines of each ten-unit increment on the gauge. Although this takes some practice, you will pick it up quickly.

7. As you continue deflating the cuff, you will soon hear the onset of clear regular tapping noises that gradually increase in intensity. When you hear the **first** of these tapping sounds, note the reading on the dial. This is your *systolic pressure*. (If you miss hearing this first beat, do not reinflate the cuff in the middle of this whole process. Instead, deflate the cuff entirely, wait about a minute, then start again.)

8. Continue to decrease the cuff pressure at the constant rate of 2 to 3 mm Hg per second. Soon, the sounds will become muffled (they may even briefly disappear), followed by the onset of loud, regular knocking sounds that gradually fade out. At the moment that all sound disappears, note the gauge reading. This is your *diastolic pressure*. Then, open the metal valve completely, allowing all remaining pressure out of the cuff and releasing the pressure on your arm. (If you miss taking a reading at the point at which all sound vanishes, do not reinflate the cuff in the midst of this process and try to take a measurement. Let all the air out of the cuff, wait a minute, then repeat the measurement process.)

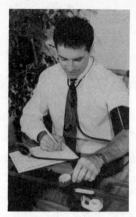

Record your systolic and diastolic pressure

9. Record your systolic and diastolic pressure. For example, if you heard the first regular beat at 125 and all sound disappeared at 85, you would record 125/85.

10. Repeat steps 5 through 9 twice. Then calculate the averages of your systolic and diastolic readings by adding all the systolic readings and dividing by the number of measurements. For example, if your systolic readings are 120, 130 and 125:

120 + 130 + 125 = 375

375 divided by 3 = 125

Enter 125 as your average systolic reading. Follow the same process to determine your average diastolic measurement. Enter these average readings in your Daily Blood Pressure log (on page 57). Remember to pause briefly between measurements to allow your circulation to return to normal. Raising the arm (with the cuff on it) above your head will rapidly restore normal circulation. It is particularly important to take three blood pressure readings using this process if your blood pressure tends to vary from reading to reading within a short time interval (labile blood pressure), or if your initial blood pressure values are higher than you had expected. When you are first learning to take your blood pressure, repeated measurements also increase your familiarity and comfort with the measurement process.

KEEPING A DAILY BLOOD PRESSURE LOG TO CHART YOUR PROGRESS

Just as captains take their bearings and keep a daily log to stay on course and steer their ship safely toward their port of destination, so should you keep a Daily Blood Pressure log to help you stay on course as you progress toward normalizing your blood pressure and reducing and eliminating your need for antihypertensive medications.

A sample Daily Blood Pressure log is shown on page 57. Each day, before and after at least one of your two relaxation sessions, take and record your blood pressure, pulse, hand or foot temperature (an objective indicator of depth of relaxation, which is discussed more fully in Chapter 7), and subjective level of tension or relaxation. Because blood pressure can fluctuate at different times of the day, be consistent about recording the results of your practice at either your earlier or later sessions. (Some people keep records of both sessions each day; if you make that choice, keep separate charts for each session.)

Over a period of weeks, you will begin to see trends in the direction of your blood pressure, which will become particularly evident as you calculate your weekly and monthly before-session blood pressure averages.

At the top of the Daily Blood Pressure log, record your name and the name of your physician, since you will be reviewing your log with your doctor for the purpose of medication changes. Enter your practice session number, the day of the week, and the calendar date that you conduct the measurements. Take your blood pressure both **before** and **after** your relaxation session, and record these readings. Do the same with your pulse rate and hand (or foot) temperature. Place an *H* or an *F* alongside the temperature reading to indicate whether it is a hand or foot measurement.

Next, rate the depth of your tension or relaxation. Just how tense or relaxed did you feel before and then after your session? Make your evaluation on a −10 to +10 scale, where +10 represents feeling completely relaxed, −10 represents feeling totally tense, +1 slightly relaxed, and −1 slightly tense.

In the next column, record your weight. Do this at least once a week, since weight changes can influence blood pressure. To be consistent, weigh yourself first thing in the morning, before breakfast. Also, whenever any changes occur in the antihypertensive medications you are on—including the kinds of medication, the dosage, and the times you take them—make a note of this information. It is important to keep track of all adjustments since they may affect your blood pressure readings. If you are on antihypertensive medication, your objective is to keep your blood pressure at or preferably below 140/90 mm Hg while your doctor gradually reduces your intake of these drugs. As your reliance on medications declines, your blood pressure measurements may remain at their current level, continue to drop, or even temporarily rise before declining again.

Also, because of the side effects and long-term risks that can be associated with medication use, your doctor may decide that you are better off taking less or no medication, even if it means having a slightly higher blood pressure without it (although still below 140/90). His or her decision will take into account how many other cardiovascular risk factors you have and the side effects you may be experiencing.

HART DAILY BLOOD PRESSURE LOG: CHARTING YOUR PROGERESS

NAME _____

PHYSICIAN _____

Starting Medication   Dosage   Time

Session Number	Day of the Week	Date	Blood Pressure Before sys	dias	After sys	dias	Pulse Before sys	After dias	Temperature Before	After H = hand F = foot	Subjective Level of Relaxation Tension −10 0 +10 Before	After	Weight	Medication Changes Name	Dosage	Time	Insights and Observation
	Week Average																
	Week Average																
	Week Average																
	Week Average																
	Monthly Average																

NOTE: For enlarged, two-page spread of this chart, see Appendix 11, pp. 252-253.

Next, keep track of other medications you may be taking for disorders unrelated to your high blood pressure. Note any changes that occur in your intake of these drugs.

Finally, in the *Insights and Observations* column, write down pertinent details about your life, such as any particular stress you may be experiencing or how you are feeling. This column is extremely important because it gives you clues as to what might be influencing your blood pressure so that you can make adjustments to bring your readings down. Problems in interpersonal relationships, career moves, and pressures at work can all have an effect on your blood pressure. In some people, blood pressure rises in response to irritation, anger, impatience, or anxiety. In others, blood pressure fluctuates in response to changes in diet, exercise, consumption of alcoholic beverages, weight changes, sleep disturbances, or travel.

You can't be absolutely certain of a causal relationship between your blood pressure and these influences—for example, there is no way to know for sure that emotional upsets or a high-salt meal make your hypertension worse. Nevertheless, you can look for patterns, and the *Insight* column will help you do that. One participant in the HART Program noticed that his blood pressure rose when he didn't get enough sleep. Another patient's blood pressure declined when he exercised regularly. Still another noted that his blood pressure increased when he was having interpersonal problems. This type of information can guide you in cultivating behavior that may contribute to normalizing your hypertension.

At the end of each week, calculate your weekly blood pressure averages by adding up all the systolic figures for the week, and dividing this number by the number of entries (preferably between five and seven). Do the same with the diastolic numbers.

After every four weeks of practice, determine your monthly before-session blood pressure averages. Add up the weekly systolic pressure and divide by the number of entries (four). This is your monthly systolic blood pressure average. Do the same with your weekly average diastolic readings.

CHECK YOUR TECHNIQUE WITH YOUR HEALTH CARE PROVIDER

In the upcoming days and weeks, as you become familiar with the ten-step process for monitoring your blood pressure, keep the instructions nearby so you can refer to them as needed. In Appendix I of the book, you will find another copy of the instructions, which you can conveniently photocopy.

Once you have a basic familiarity with taking your blood pressure, bring your measurement device and the instructions for taking your blood pressure to your next doctor's visit. If you have no plans to see your doctor soon, schedule a visit to ask for your physician's support as you engage in this program and to get your technique checked. When you make the appointment, explain that you need assistance with measuring your blood pressure so the doctor or nurse will set aside the time required. Ask your healthcare provider to help you refine your technique if necessary, because you want to make certain that you are taking your blood pressure accurately.

At the HART Institute, the project staff carefully checks each participants' blood pressure measurements for accuracy, using a dual training stethoscope with two sets of ear pieces (available at medical supply stores), which enables both patient and healthcare provider to hear the same sounds as they watch the gauge. The staff works together with the patient until each hears, sees, and records the same blood pressure reading three times in a row. To be considered accurate, patient and provider should agree that the three measurements are within 4 mm Hg of one another.

CHECK YOUR EQUIPMENT PERIODICALLY

During that same visit to your physician's office, you may wish to check the results you obtained from your blood pressure equipment against those from your doctor's mercury column device. This will ensure that your own equipment is working correctly. It is important to periodically check to make sure your sphygmomanometer is calibrated (adjusted) accurately and that there are no leaks or tears in the tubing that will interfere with accurate readings. In aneroid models, regularly check the needle on the gauge to make sure it is at zero when the cuff is deflated. If it is not, send it back to the factory to be recalibrated. If your model needs worn parts replaced, they can usually be ordered. As a general guideline, if you start getting consistent readings that vary considerably from your customary ones, check your equipment; it may be time for recalibrating or replacement.

TROUBLESHOOTING COMMON PROBLEMS & ERRORS

As you fine-tune your blood pressure measurement technique, be aware that there are several common sources of error in this process:

You may be somewhat nervous during your first few attempts at taking your blood pressure. As a result, your blood pressure readings may be higher than you anticipate. This is a common problem. To counteract it, take a few long and deep breaths and relax. As you master the basics with a few days of practice, you will gradually become more comfortable and at ease with the technique. Also, remind yourself that you are participating in this program because your blood pressure is high and that it **will** come down as you practice your relaxation techniques.

You may have difficulty locating your brachial artery, either due to lack of experience or because the pulsations are somewhat weak. Or perhaps you are not probing in the right place on your arm. Often, a brief period of exercise will increase the pulse strength, making it easier to find. If you still can't find it, ask your healthcare provider for help.

If you miss hearing the first regular tapping sound of your systolic blood pressure, or regularly hear and read it as lower than it actually is, try inflating the pressure in the cuff higher, and then letting the air out more slowly so you have more control. Make sure you inflate your cuff to 210 mm Hg (or at least 30 points above your systolic pressure, whichever is greater), and then carefully deflate it at a slow, steady rate, allowing the hand of the dial to pulse twice within every 10 mm Hg. By releasing the valve of the gauge slowly, you will have more control, so the dial will not descend too rapidly.

You might have some difficulty hearing the very soft, final sounds just before obtaining your diastolic blood pressure. To determine your diastolic reading, you need to hear that last sound and then note your pressure reading, which corresponds to the first moment of silence. If you aren't precise in picking out when sound completely disappears, you will arrive at an inaccurate reading. This is a learning process; be patient, make sure the stethoscope is directly over the brachial artery, and always conduct your measurement in a quiet environment. If you have a hearing problem, it is better to use an automatic blood pressure device.

When reading the blood pressure dial, you may have difficulty seeing each measurement "freshly." Instead, your reading is colored by what you **expect** to see or hear. You will increase your accuracy if you cultivate a "beginner's mind." Drop your expectations of what your blood pressure should be and see it anew each time you take it.

Another common source of inaccuracy is rounding off your reading. If the hand on the dial is at 91 mm Hg, you need to record 91, not 90, to be accurate. Practice reading and recording the exact placement of the dial so your Daily Blood Pressure Log will provide you with accurate, high-quality information.

TEACH A FRIEND OR FAMILY MEMBER

Teaching a family member or a friend how to take your blood pressure—or, for that matter, how to take their own—is a good way to increase your ease with the measurement process. HART patients have gotten their mates, children, secretaries, and friends to participate. This is a way of demystifying blood pressure for the important people in your life, while providing them with skills they can also use to monitor a vital sign important to their own health. By learning the technique with another person, you'll also tend to defuse any stress you're feeling in trying to measure your own blood pressure.

If you still need help with your blood pressure measurement technique, go back to your physician, or to the nurse or healthcare technician in the doctor's office. He or she can guide you through the entire process, troubleshooting as you go along.

MONITORING YOUR PULSE

Your pulse is the rhythmic throbbing at your wrist, the side of your neck, or anywhere on the body where an artery comes close to the skin's surface. It is a reflection of your heart rate. Each time your heart contracts, ejecting blood from the left ventricle into the arteries, a wave of pressure moves through the arteries and causes the expansion and contraction that we detect as a pulse. By taking your pulse, you can determine the number of times your heart beats per minute.

As previously described, the formula for blood pressure,

blood pressure = cardiac output × peripheral resistance

indicates that the heart rate—since it affects cardiac output—is an important factor influencing blood pressure. Of course, a number of factors can make your heart rate rise, including exercise, fighting off an infection, food allergies, or stress. A persistently elevated pulse can also be an indicator that your heart is working too hard, which can contribute to the onset and maintenance of high blood pressure. **Heart rate is closely connected with high blood pressure. A lower pulse rate is generally consistent with decreased blood pressure.**

A normal adult resting heart rate ranges from about 60 to 90 beats per minute (athletes may have a resting range as low as 40 to 60 beats). In this program, you will want to see a decrease in your pulse rate after your relaxation practice, as well as over the long term of this program if it is anything but low when you start. If you can lower your pulse, this in turn can contribute to a decline in your blood pressure. A lower resting heart rate in adults is also associated with a more efficient heart; this is because the lower your resting pulse, the less hard your heart has to work. Of course, pulse rates vary from moment to moment, and just as your pulse might speed up in response to stimulants such as caffeine, cigarettes, diet pills, and decongestants, it will slow down when you take medications like digitalis or beta-blockers.

You will also probably find that your pulse rate declines after your relaxation practice—but not always. There may be fluctuations due to stress or other factors in your life. If you have been taking medications such as beta blockers that keep your pulse low, you might see some increase as you taper off your antihypertensive medications. A program of regular exercise can help bring your pulse down. We are interested in long-term trends, and over time, you will want to be able to bring a high pulse rate down. Naturally, as your pulse rate stabilizes at a lower plateau, you may see smaller declines after each relaxation session.

TAKING YOUR PULSE

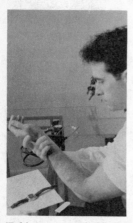

Taking your radial pulse

Whenever you measure your blood pressure, you should also measure and record your pulse rate on your log sheet. You will need a watch with a second hand or a digital display. The most convenient places to measure your pulse are over the radial artery on your wrist, or over the carotid artery at the side of your neck.

To locate your *radial pulse,* place the index and middle fingers of your right hand on the underside of your left wrist, just below the base of your thumb. Using the flat of your fingers, not the tips, press gently but firmly until you feel the rhythmic beat of your pulse. While you could count each beat of your pulse for 60 seconds to determine your pulse rate, it is more efficient to count the number of beats for 15 seconds and multiply by 4.

If you prefer, you can perform this measurement over your *carotid artery.* Place your index and middle fingers in the soft indentation on the side of your neck, right beneath your jaw bone.

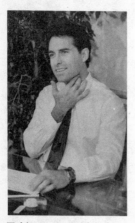

Taking your pulse from the carotid artery

Again, press gently but firmly until you feel your pulse. It is best not to use your thumb, which has its own pulse, or to press so strongly that you interfere with the pulse. Pressing too hard over the carotid pulse can slow beats by three to four per minute.

Even if you just can't seem to find your pulse, rest assured that it's there. Quite commonly, people find and lose their pulse a few times during the learning process. Exercising briefly will strengthen your pulse, making it easier to find. Once you become efficient at this process, monitoring your pulse will take just fifteen seconds—hands on!

CHAPTER · 7

_____

Starting Your Biobehavioral Program:
Temperature Feedback and Autogenics

*I had heard about biofeedback. . . I can now say categorically
that it works. From the moment I started the HART
Program, I could see slow, steady improvement as my blood
pressure went down; at points when the stress in my life
increased, I could see it take a turn up. But always, I could
see the positive training effect before and after relaxation.*

> —ROBERT
> Attorney
> HART participant

IT IS TIME to begin learning the skills of the biobehavioral core of the
HART Program. Biobehavioral treatment consists of regularly practicing deep psychophysiological relaxation, assisted by temperature feedback, in your daily life.

This chapter focuses on temperature feedback and autogenic
phrases—the first two in a series of six self-regulatory skills which, when
regularly practiced, have helped many individuals bring their hypertension under control and eliminate or greatly reduce their need for
antihypertensive medication. It also includes recommendations for op-
timizing your relaxation practice. In the subsequent chapters, you will
learn the other HART biobehavioral techniques: Systematic Muscular
Relaxation, Three-Part Complete Breathing, Imaging, and Constant
Instant Practice.

To maximize your results, it is important for you to take the time to
learn and integrate each of these skills into twice-daily, fifteen-minute
relaxation practice sessions. Each technique is a self-regulatory process
that can assist you in learning to orchestrate your mind, body, and
breathing to achieve a state of deep psychophysiological relaxation.
While you need to pay attention to each skill during the initial learning
stages, it will soon become second nature for you to relax deeply and
manage stress more effectively.

HOW THE PROGRAM WORKS

Before you actually get started, let's take a moment to recap and elaborate on some of the most relevant rationale for this program's effectiveness. Earlier in the book, you read about some of your body's autonomic functions, including breathing mechanisms, heart rate, body temperature, and blood pressure. These have traditionally been considered automatic, physiological processes that were regulated by the part of the involuntary nervous system thought to be outside your conscious influence or control. However, more than two decades ago, scientific developments leading to the advent of the new field of biobehavioral treatment—utilizing biofeedback and behavioral change—demonstrated that voluntary control of many physiological functions **is** learnable. Feeback-assisted relaxation training, aided by instruments such as thermometers, can enable us to gain control over autonomically-regulated bodily processes. The instruments function as mirrors, "feeding back" second-by-second information about silent, internal biological activity—hence the term *biofeedback*. As they provide us with information about our ongoing physiological functions such as body temperature or heart rate, for instance, we can gradually learn—through a process of experimentation or trial-and-error—subtle ways to mentally influence and redirect our biological processes in the direction of better health.

Though biofeedback is a relatively new science, feedback itself is really nothing new; in fact, it has been integral to almost everything you've learned throughout your life. Dr. Barbara Brown, a pioneer in biofeedback research, has suggested that if you'd like to know if voluntary control of autonomic processes is possible, just look in the mirror and wink. You might remember as a child learning to wink by imitating a parent or practicing in a mirror. While the blinking action of both eyes is an ongoing, autonomically-regulated process that keeps the eyeballs lubricated, blinking just one eye is an acquired skill that takes practice to learn. If you can wink, you already have experience learning to self-regulate an autonomically-regulated process.

Sports are another example in which feedback enables you to learn a new skill. When you pick up a tennis racket and hit the ball over the net, for example, you probably become a little better with each successive week of practice, by using various visual and sensory information: such input as the speed the ball is moving, how close you are to hitting it, and whether you need to swing a bit higher or lower, faster of slower. This kind of information is internalized by your brain and central nervous system and is used to make adjustments in the actions of nerve cells in the muscles. This, in turn, increases the fine-tuned control of your next swing until you are finally hitting the ball accurately and consistently, without giving it much thought at all. Some people call it "eye-hand coordination;" but more appropriately, it might be called "mind-body coordination."

For more formal biofeedback training, a clinician might attach a set of electronic sensors to your body to monitor functions like skin temperature, muscle tension, and heart rate. Then you might be led through a series of relaxation techniques and be asked to imagine yourself relaxing in a comfortable and beautiful place of your choice. As you do so, the dials and meters in front of you may begin to show gradual and then substantial changes, including a rise in your finger temperature, a decrease in muscle tension, and a deceleration of your heart rate. These changes occur as you receive feedback from the instrumentation and learn to modify your internal sensations, feelings, breathing patterns, images, and thoughts in the direction of autonomic and muscular relaxation. It is a remarkable process and a clear example of the mastery you can develop over your mind-body. In fact, not only can we learn to change our heart rate or temperature, but if accurate feedback is provided, we can influence our physiology so specifically that we can influence the acidity in our stomach and the wave patterns in our brain, and even activate the firing of just a single neuron in our spine. Dr. Barbara Brown has stated that our self-regulatory capacity may be limited only by our biomedical instrumentation; if we have the instrumentation to provide us with feedback on a specific physiological function, we can learn to voluntarily control this function.

In essence, biofeedback training gives the conscious parts of your brain information about functions of which you are normally unaware. When that happens, you create a two-way line of communication or biocybernetic loop between your brain and the physiological process you want to influence, eliminating the chasm between voluntary and involuntary.

Where does this self-regulatory capacity come from? As we discussed in Chapter 3, it lies in the complicated neurophysiological network that intricately links body and mind. Even when we're not conscious of it, our brain is continuously controlling many bodily processes. We may not understand how it happens, particularly because it is outside our conscious awareness, but every mental event has a corresponding physiological event—that is, every thought and every emotion trigger physiological changes, and every physiological change affects our thoughts and feelings.

Fortunately, we do not need to fully understand or be aware of every neurophysiological process that occurs when our mind exerts such control over autonomic functions. More than anything, we need to recognize that once we become consciously aware of a physiological process through biofeedback, we can learn to re-regulate it.

As you practice feedback-assisted relaxation in the weeks ahead, you will be developing strategies to decrease the overactivity of the sympathetic branch of your Autonomic Nervous System (ANS). By regulating the warmth of your hand, the depth and rate of respiration, and the degree of muscle tension or relaxation, you will be moving towards greater autonomic balance, lower blood pressure, and better health.

With practice, you will eventually be able to elicit a deeply relaxed state rapidly **without** using the feedback device. That is why regular practice is so important. By mastering the relaxation and self-regulation skills, you will be internalizing the learning processes and they will become natural and self-perpetuating.

In learning to regulate your blood pressure, you do not need to give any more attention to the complex, underlying physiological processes involved than you did when, for example, you learned to ride a bike. You will gradually learn and master your self-regulation skills, and as that happens, they will always be there for you to use.

In addition to seeing your blood pressure decrease, you may be pleasantly surprised by how much better you feel as you take time out of each day to relax and break the stress cycle. When you remove the effects of chronic, stress-related overactivation of body-mind, your own intrinsic capacity for self-healing becomes operative, resulting in increased psychophysiological health and balance.

TEMPERATURE AS AN INDICATOR OF AUTONOMIC RELAXATION

Let's spend a few moments examining your hand temperature more closely. Nearly everyone knows that the normal body temperature is 98.6 degrees Farenheit. Yet most people give very little thought to their hand or foot temperature, which is usually lower than their core body temperature.

While your core temperature generally does not vary more than a few degrees from 98.6, there can be a much wider range of peripheral readings—that is, the temperature of your hands and feet—sometimes with swings as great as 25 degrees. When patients first begin working with temperature feedback, they can tell whether their hands feel warm or cold, but they usually can't pinpoint their hand temperature to within even five degrees of accuracy. That's why a thermometer or other accurate measuring device is so essential to your success with this program.

High blood pressure, remember, is considered a vasoconstrictive disorder. When the fight-or-flight mechanism is set into motion, sympathetic activity increases. As that happens, there is a response within the vessels (or arterioles) that supply blood to your body periphery. The smooth muscles in the vessel walls react to this sympathetic arousal by contracting or vasoconstricting (vaso means vessel). You may experience the resulting decrease in blood circulation as a cooling of your hands.

Take a moment right now to touch your fingertips to your cheek. Do they feel warm or cold? If you're calm and relaxed, your hands will probably be warm to the touch. However, if you're under stress, they will probably be cooler.

A decrease in your peripheral body temperature indicates an increase in the activity of your sympathetic nervous system; by contrast, when your peripheral temperature rises, your sympathetic nervous system is becoming increasingly relaxed. As this latter process occurs, the blood vessel walls dilate and blood flow increases, which you experience as greater warmth. At the same time, your pulse rate declines—and your blood pressure may decrease as well. Interestingly, this is similar to the sympathetic deactivation achieved by a class of hypertension medications called the *sympathetic inhibitors*.

Temperature feedback is in fact a key to normalizing your blood pressure. A study by Dr. M. Hartfield examined the effectiveness of a basic biobehavioral protocol in the treatment of essential hypertension in two groups of patients. Only one of these groups used temperature feedback as part of their program; the other group underwent the same training but without the temperature feedback component. The group of patients who used temperature feedback normalized their blood pressure, while the others, who did not use temperature feedback, were not able to reduce their blood pressure. In this study, temperature feedback was the key to successfully normalizing blood pressure.

Specifically, the HART Program will ask you to use temperature feedback to warm your hands to 95.5–96 degrees, and your feet to about 93 degrees for at least a 10-minute period during each of your twice-a-day sessions. Warming your hands and feet to these levels and for this amount of time provides an objective indicator that you have decreased the activity of your sympathetic nervous system, vasodilated your body periphery, and attained a state of deep, autonomic psychophysiological relaxation—all of which contribute to regulating your blood pressure. Remember the *ART* in HART stands for Autonomic Relaxation Treatment. You are literally relaxing the sympathetic branch of your ANS.

TEMPERATURE FEEDBACK TRAINING: GETTING STARTED

In this section, as well as in your ensuing relaxation sessions, you will need a device to monitor the temperature of your hands. Small thermometers or biotic bands are inexpensive and work quite well, as does the more costly digital thermistor, an electronic device with a digital display. Small thermometers can be purchased at hardware stores. Biotic bands and digital thermistors can be bought at biomedical supply houses. Both devices are effective; however, some patients decide to invest in the more expensive digital equipment because they find the numerical display easier to read.

Once you have a thermometer or other temperature feedback device in hand, take a few minutes to do the following brief process, in order to begin to explore how feelings, thoughts, and images can influence your hand temperature. To begin, attach your temperature monitoring device to your finger. If you are using a simple thermometer, tape the red ball onto the pad of a finger on your dominant hand—that is, if you are right-handed, place it on a finger of your right hand; if you are left-handed, use a finger of your left hand. The red ball needs to be placed snugly to ensure good contact, but not so tightly that you constrict circulation. If your finger or toe turns white, you have applied it too tightly.

If you are using a biotic band, attach it securely around your finger, ensuring that its face is in contact with the pad of your finger and not over the nail. For digital thermistors, attach the temperature sensor to the pad of your finger. Take a moment to familiarize yourself with your temperature feedback device.

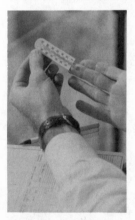

Sit back in a comfortable chair and give your temperature device a few seconds to register your hand temperature and stabilize there. Record this temperature reading, which is referred to as your starting or baseline temperature. To ensure that you are monitoring your actual hand temperature, keep the palm of your hand up and your fingers uncurled; if you were to place the hand—and the temperature-sensitive part of your thermometer—against another part of your body, the reading would be warmer than your actual peripheral hand temperature.

Attach your thermometer or temperature monitoring device to your finger

Once you have recorded the temperature, relax, take a few long, deep breaths, and recall a situation in which you felt particularly at ease and very relaxed. For a few minutes, vividly relive or recreate this experience in your mind's eye as if you were actually there right now. Allow your sense of ease and relaxation to deepen. Intermittently, look at your hand temperature. As you relax more deeply, the temperature will probably increase.

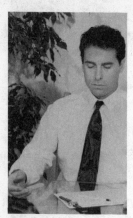

Relax

When you have completed this process, check your temperature again and record the reading. How much has it changed? Do you feel differently than before? If you'd like, watch your temperature device and allow yourself to relax even more completely. See if, through increasing your sense of relaxation, you can raise the temperature even a little more. You are now beginning to learn to use temperature feedback to assist you in warming your hands and deepening your relaxation.

Next, close your eyes once more and think of an event or circumstance you find moderately stressful; for example, coping with bumper-to-bumper traffic during rush hour as you become increasingly late for an important appointment or giving a presentation. Whatever image you choose, focus on it for a minute or two, seeing and feeling it as clearly as possible. Then open your eyes, and check and record your hand temperature again.

Did your thoughts and feelings have an effect on your temperature? Was it different when you imagined an experience in which you felt at ease, compared to one in which you felt stressed? If so, this is a clear and simple demonstration of the body-mind connection, a process which will become clearer as you practice feedback-assisted deep relaxation.

Changes in the temperature of your body's periphery (both hands and feet) are mediated almost solely by the sympathetic branch of your ANS. This is the part of the nervous system that plays such a critical role in your body's response to stress. Thus, your hand and foot temperature are excellent indicators of whether you are relaxed or under stress. Once you are able to raise your hand temperature to 95.5 degrees, it is time to shift the focus of your sessions from warming your hands to warming your feet. To do this, move the thermometer or thermistor to your foot, taping it onto the pad of your big toe, again on your dominant side. While warming your feet can take a bit more time and experimentation to learn, considerably more of your total body vasculature is located in your legs and feet. Be patient. If you can learn to warm your hands, you can learn to warm your feet. As you learn and practice the techniques of the program, be aware how subtle

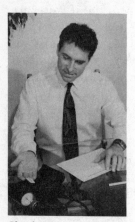

Check your temperature again and record it

changes in your thoughts, feelings, emotions, and breathing can significantly raise your temperature. Temperature feedback will let you know when your warming and relaxation strategies are on target.

WHAT IS AUTOGENICS?

Dr. Kenneth Pelletier, an internationally acknowledged authority on the prevention and treatment of stress-related disorders, calls autogenic training one of the most comprehensive and successful Western deep-relaxation techniques. *Autogenics* comes from the Greek root words *auto* and *genous,* which together mean "self-generation" or "self-creation."

Although not widely known in the U.S., autogenic training is highly respected and has a long history of use in Europe. It was developed in 1932 by psychiatrist Johannes H. Schultz, who began using it successfully for the treatment of high blood pressure, digestive disorders and musculoskeletal problems. Since then, its therapeutic applications have expanded to include a wide variety of cardiovascular, respiratory, endocrine, gastrointestinal, metabolic, and sleep disorders.

One of the basic assumptions behind autogenics is that humans are innately equipped with "self-regulatory brain mechanisms" that maintain a dynamic balance or homeostasis in all our bodily functions. When this homeostasis is disrupted, our self-regulating mechanisms have the capability of restoring a healthy equilibrium, whether by calming an escalated heart rate, lowering elevated blood pressure, or healing an ulcer.

Ron, a slim young man in his twenties, represents an excellent example of the usefulness of autogenics. Ron was planning to drop out of the university because he was having bouts of tachycardia, or sudden escalations of his heart rate, which had become uncontrollable. This was understandably quite frightening for him, and would cause incapacitating anxiety attacks.

Ron's regular physician had been unable to help him, so Ron decided to explore autogenic training, based on the premise that his tachycardia was stress-related and that he could use it to re-regulate his heart rate.

Within months, Ron had indeed learned to bring his heart rate under control through daily practice with autogenic phrases. His tachycardia disappeared, he was able to stay in school, and he graduated and went on to a satisfying career.

Getting Started with Autogenic Phrases

A component of autogenic training is the use of autogenic phrases, which are verbal formulas that, when practiced regularly, can elicit a desired psychophysiological state. These phrases promote a deep state of relaxation and allow you to consciously or voluntarily control physiological functions such as temperature, breathing, heart rate, and circulation.

Through autogenics, you can influence physiological functions by inwardly repeating phrases that describe desired psychophysiological states. In tandem with temperature feedback, the phrases are important tools for deeply relaxing your autonomic nervous system and normalizing your blood pressure.

As you may recall, stress-related disorders tend to develop because of a prolonged overactivation of the body-mind. Even while you sleep, your body, mind, and emotions can be exceedingly active. Through the use of autogenic phrases, you can bring about a state of quietness that is important to regaining the state of homeostasis necessary for self-healing to occur. Dr. Elmer Green and Alyce Green of the Menninger Foundation have compared trying to program the mind/body while it is not quiet to attempting to record with a tape machine that is set for 'playback.' Until the machine is placed in the 'record' setting, it will not record. Our minds and bodies, according to the Greens, appear to be in the playback mode a good deal of the time, even while asleep. They observe that we can even worry more while dreaming than while we are awake.

Autogenics, added the Greens, enable patients with hypertension to develop "the ability to turn off chronic tension in the sympathetic nervous system (the 'fight-or-flight' system) and helps develop a more relaxed style of living."

While practicing the autogenic phrases, you may experience feelings of inner quiet, heaviness, and warmth. These are subjective indicators of a deeply relaxed state of body and mind. The quietness correlates with the calming of mental activity and a state of relaxed awareness; the heaviness with deep muscular relaxation; and the warmth with the increased blood flow resulting from the vasodilation of the peripheral arteries. These sensations correspond to a state of equilibrium or homeostasis within the body-mind.

This section does not emphasize trying to control the natural system, but rather helping natural systems use their inherent potential to regulate themselves more fully.

When you first start using the autogenic phrases, you may want to tape-record the entire set and practice as you play them back. Or, if you prefer, you can alternate between reading each phrase, then closing your eyes and experiencing the changes described by that phrase.

Whichever option you choose, remember to read the phrases in a calm, deliberate, relaxed manner. The quality, tempo, and tone of your voice can either encourage or interfere with your relaxation. Cultivate a pleasant mid-range tone rather than a high-pitched one, and a moderate pace rather than a rapid rate of speech. This will contribute significantly to the ease and depth of your relaxation. Before you begin your first session, however, be sure to read to the end of this chapter, so you will have all the information you need to make the most effective use of your autogenics relaxation practice.

USING AUTOGENIC PHRASES EFFECTIVELY

1. If you are reading the phrases rather than listening to them from a tape, be sure to keep your gaze soft and passive rather than overly active. If you strain your eyes, you will inadvertently contract some of the muscles that you want to relax. After scanning each phrase, close your eyes and experience the changes taking place that are described by that phrase.
2. With each phrase, see and feel the part of your body that is being described. This establishes a connection between your awareness and the part of you you are concentrating on. Throughout the exercise, keep a steady flow of images, feelings, and bodily sensations. This will encourage your body and mind to be most responsive to the changes you want to make.
3. Experiment with various techniques for repeating the autogenic phrases to yourself. After listening to a phrase, repeat it silently or out loud; or, if you are a very visual person, you might want to imagine the words written. Find out what works best for you.
4. When using temperature feedback with autogenics phrases, periodically note and record your hand temperature to see what phrases show the greatest increase in temperature. Also, be aware of the particular images, feelings, and sensations you experience with these phrases; these can increase your body peripheral temperature.

YOUR AUTOGENICS AND TEMPERATURE FEEDBACK SESSION

The autogenic phrases used in the HART Program are adaptations of a short form of autogenic training developed by Dr. Elmer Green, Alyce Green and Dr. Dale Walters at the Voluntary Controls program of the Menninger Foundation.

To begin your session, gently close your eyes and relax. Then move through the complete list of phrases, repeating each of them two or three times, pausing between each repetition for a few seconds to allow your mind-body to respond.

Remember to use temperature feedback during your session, glancing at your hand temperature to objectively note the effect of your moment-by-moment practice. In later sessions, you might use temperature feedback more sparingly. Record or ask a friend or family member to record your changes in hand temperature as you practice the following set of autogenic phrases.

AUTOGENIC PHRASES

Hand Temperature

_____ Starting Temperature

Relaxation Phrases

_____ I feel very quiet.

_____ I am beginning to feel quiet and relaxed.

_____ My feet feel heavy, relaxed, and comfortable.

_____ My ankles, knees, and hips feel heavy, relaxed, and comfortable.

_____ My solar plexus and the whole central region of my body feel relaxed and quiet.

_____ My hands, arms, and shoulders feel heavy, quiet, relaxed, and comfortable.

_____ My neck, jaws, and forehead feel relaxed. They feel comfortable and quiet.

_____ My whole body feels quiet, heavy, comfortable, and relaxed.

_____ For the next minute, continue focusing on this experience of quiet, heaviness, comfort, and relaxation.

Warmth Phrases

_____ I am quite relaxed.

_____ My arms and hands are heavy, comfortable, and warm.

_____ I feel inwardly quiet.

_____ My whole body is relaxed and comfortable, and my hands are relaxed and warm.

_____ Warmth is flowing into my hands. They are warm, warm.

_____ I can feel the warmth flowing down my arms and into my hands.

_____ For the next minutes, continue feeling quiet, relaxed, and warm.

Inner Quietness and Calming Phrases

_____ My entire body feels quiet, comfortable, and relaxed.

_____ My mind is quiet and calm.

_____ I withdraw my thoughts from the surroundings and I feel inwardly serene and still.

_____ My thoughts are turned inward and I am quiet, at ease, and calm.

_____ Deep within my mind, I can see and feel myself as relaxed, comfortable, serene, and still.

_____ I am alert, yet in an easy, quiet, and inward way.

_____ My mind is calm, quiet, and serene.

_____ I feel inwardly quiet.

Energizing Phrases

_____ I reactivate my body with a deep breath and the following phrases: I feel life, light, and energy flowing through my feet, legs, thighs, hips, solar plexus, chest, hands, arms, shoulders, neck, and head.

_____ My autogenics session for relaxation, warmth, and quiet is now complete. I feel relaxed, inwardly quiet, healthy, energized, and alive.

_____ FINAL TEMPERATURE   _____ HIGHEST TEMPERATURE

REFINING YOUR SKILLS BY REFLECTING ON YOUR SESSION

As with mastering any other skill, learning how to relax and warm your hands takes time and practice. You can speed up the process, however, by identifying the particular images, sensations, emotions, and thoughts that most effectively warm your hands, and using these experiences during your practice.

The following Temperature Feedback-Assisted Relaxation inventory can help you discover what works best for you. It will also give you an opportunity to look at your practice more objectively to identify and solve any problems.

TEMPERATURE FEEDBACK-ASSISTED RELAXATION INVENTORY

Following one of your relaxation sessions each day, take a few minutes to learn from your experience by answering the following questions:

Note your before-relaxation-session
    hand (foot) temperature ____
Note your after-relaxation-session
    hand (foot) temperature ____

1. Were you able to relax? If not, what seemed to interfere?

2. If you did relax and warm your hands (feet), what phrases helped you the most? Place a star by these phrases on your list.

3. When using the phrases that were most effective in deepening your relaxation and increasing your hand (foot) warmth, did you establish contact with the part of the body described in the phrase by:
   a. sensing or feeling that part?
   b. seeing or visualizing that part?
   c. both (a) and (b)?

4. Were you able to feel the following changes:
   a. Warmth: Definitely   Moderately   Slightly   Not at All
   b. Flushing: Definitely   Moderately   Slightly   Not at All
   c. Throbbing/Pulsating: Definitely   Moderately
       Slightly   Not at All

5. Describe the physical sensations, emotions, or images that accompanied the phrases you found most effective for relaxing and increasing your hand temperature.
   Physical sensations:
   Emotions:
   Images:

6. During this session, did your mind wander:
   a. not at all?
   b. a little?
   c. a lot?

7. During this session, did you:
   a. feel relaxed but alert?
   b. feel drowsy?
   c. fall asleep?

8. Did your blood pressure and/or pulse decrease after your session?

OPTIMIZING THE BENEFITS OF YOUR RELAXATION PRACTICE

The following recommendations will assist you in making the most of your relaxation practice:

1. **Practice in a quiet place with subdued lighting, a comfortable temperature, and minimal distractions.** This is an important time you are setting aside for yourself and your health, so do what you can to minimize interruptions. For example, turn your telephone answering machine on, or request that someone else answer the phone and take messages. Place a *Please Do Not Disturb* sign on your door. Ask others for their support in keeping the environment quiet.

   Subdued lighting and a comfortable temperature also adds to the effectiveness of your practice. A cool room can make it difficult for you to relax and effectively practice warming your hands. If you can't control the temperature where you are so you can relax comfortably, put on extra clothing or use a blanket.

2. **Keep your supplies at hand.** Make sure you have the supplies you'll need for self-monitoring and record-keeping, including a blood pressure measuring device, thermometer, tape, Daily Blood Pressure Log, pen or pencil, and a clock or watch with a second hand (for monitoring your pulse).

3. **Take and record measurements before and after practice.** Before and after your relaxation practice, take your blood pressure, pulse, and hand (foot) temperature, and record these measurements in your Daily Blood Pressure log.

4. **Relax in a comfortable position.** Either sit or recline in a balanced, symmetrical position. This will help your maximize your results, while also making your sessions more enjoyable. For complete relaxation, support your body as completely as possible. Also remember to loosen any tight clothing, belts, ties, and jewelry.

5. **Develop a comfortable reclining position.** This is the best position for home practice. Select a comfortable, but firm surface that will enable you to stretch out completely, such as a firm, wide couch, recliner, bed, or foam mat.

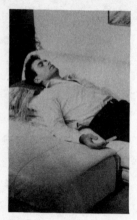

Reclining with cushions and towel roll under head and chest—additional support under knees

While resting on your back, place your legs hip-distance apart and relaxed, with your feet gently inclined outward. Extend your arms comfortably alongside but not touching your torso. Place your palms up, with your fingers relaxed and apart. Position your arms and legs symmetrically and evenly apart on both sides of your body. Make sure your spine is relaxed yet straight and extended, and your head and neck are relaxed and in alignment with your spinal column (not tilted to either side). Align your trunk and shoulders, and adjust your hips and shoulders so they are parallel to one another. Gently draw the lower tips of your shoulder blades forward and allow your shoulders to relax downward (away from your ears). Note how this opens your chest and straightens your spine.

If you find it more comfortable, you may wish to use one or more cushions or a rolled towel or blanket under your head, chest, and knees. This additional support can open and ease tightness or constriction in your chest and make breathing easier (some experts have found that additional support under the head and chest during reclining relaxation can be particularly helpful for persons who suffer from abnormal heartbeats, feel heaviness or discomfort in the heart area, or have enlarged ventricle or congenital heart defects).

If you are unable to straighten your legs comfortably or if you have back problems, place a folded or rolled blanket under your knees. This releases strain on the lower back by straightening out the lumbar curve and more firmly supporting it. Once you are comfortable, tilt your forehead slightly forward. Focusing your gaze on your heart can be quite calming.

6. **Develop a comfortable sitting position.** When you're away from home—in the office, for instance—or if you tend to fall asleep when you lie down, then sitting up makes more sense. An easy chair, a recliner or a straight-backed chair will work. If you choose an easy chair, it is best to select one that's designed to fit your body. High-backed chairs or recliners allow your back, torso, and head to rest passively and be comfortably supported during the relaxation practice. When possible, use a chair in which the length of the seat is equal to the length of your thighs; this will permit your lower back to rest against the back of the

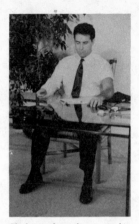

Sitting relaxation practice

chair or use a cushion behind your back for support.

In a straight-backed chair, position your back comfortably against the chair, with your spine elongated and relaxed to prevent slumping, which could impede your breathing. Slightly tilt your chin downward. Keep the back of your neck long and the front of your throat soft. Do not let your head fall so far forward that the weight of your head causes the back of your neck to feel strained. Extend your legs forward, then draw your feet back toward you until both feet are flat and well-supported by the floor. The angle between your lower legs and the floor should be more than 90 degrees. (If your feet do not reach the ground, place a phone book or other object underneath them so they are supported.)

Relax your arms on the arms of the chair, or supported alongside your body, palms up, hands and fingers relaxed and open (not in a fist).

Once you are comfortable, make sure your body is symmetrical, with your arms and feet resting equidistant apart. Keep your head aligned with your spine. To adjust your shoulders and open your chest so you do not slouch (which would compress your breathing), gently adjust the lower tips of your shoulder blades down and forward.

7. **Adopt an attitude to encourage relaxation.** Adopt an expectant yet detached attitude toward your relaxation practice. This means intending and allowing yourself to experience what takes place without being concerned or worrying about obtaining results—let the relaxing and warming take place rather than actively striving to bring about the desired changes. If you **try** to relax and raise your hand temperature, you may actually bring about the opposite result—cooling your hands and decreasing your sense of ease. By intending to relax and then being receptive and "letting it happen," the relaxation and warming will occur spontaneously, using your inherent potential for self-regulatory adjustment. Such an attitude of "quiet receptivity" or "passive volition" facilitates the cooperation with your autonomic, self-regulating system, and also helps you fine-tune your skills in this area.

8. **Practice feedback-assisted autogenics and hand-warming twice a day for the next few days to a week.** Use the entire set

of phrases for a week, then just the phrases that work best for you. Or if you prefer, develop your own phrases.

Once you feel comfortable with your autogenics practice, go on to the next chapter on breathing. By making the exercises in this and the following chapters a priority in your life, you will reap significant dividends in terms of your blood pressure and overall health.

COMMON PROBLEMS DURING RELAXATION PRACTICE

Common problems that you may encounter during your relaxation practice, including what to do about them, are described as follows:

1. **Distracting Thoughts.** Often, we are unaware just how active our minds are until we turn our focus within and begin to relax. When thoughts come up, notice them, then gently return your attention to your relaxation and warming practice. Rather than fighting or suppressing thoughts, just refocus your attention on the task at hand as rapidly as possible.

   It can be useful to view distracting thoughts as a flock of birds or butterflies flying across the screen of your mind, or as clouds dispersing in an open blue sky. If your mind keeps coming up with tasks that urgently need to be done or you catch yourself repeatedly rehashing something that concerns you, imagine symbolically placing your tasks or concerns in a jar on a mantelpiece, leaving them there until your session is done, and then picking them up and, if appropriate, attending to them at that time.

   The breathing techniques you will learn in the next chapter are also very helpful in quieting your mind so you can focus on relaxing.

2. **Feeling Drowsy or Falling Asleep.** When first starting relaxation practice, some people feel somewhat drowsy or even briefly fall asleep. With practice, however, you will develop the ability to be deeply relaxed yet alert during your relaxation session. Relaxed alertness is a regenerative state well worth cultivating.

   If you do get drowsy, practice while sitting up rather than lying down. If you still feel sleepy, your body may be telling you that you need more sleep. Getting seven or eight hours of sleep a night is important for health and longevity.

3. **Distractions in Your External Environment.** If there are many distractions in your environment, find a way to take care of them so they won't interfere with your practice. For example, if

you are bothered by traffic noise, consider using relaxing music, a soothing environmental soundtrack, or a white noise generator such as a fan to muffle the outside noise. If family members are the source of the distraction, ask for their cooperation during these brief time intervals, and let them know that these sessions are important to your health.

4. **Your Hands and Feet Become Cool Instead of Warm.** If you find that your body peripheral temperature does not change, or it cools rather than warms, check your environment. A room temperature that is too cool for comfort or is drafty, can add unneeded difficulty to your practice.

If you continue to notice your body peripheral temperature cooling rather than warming, turn this to your advantage by learning what you are doing to effectively cool your hands or feet. Specifically, be aware of your thoughts, feelings, images, and what you may be saying to yourself internally. Note whether your attitude is one of relaxed awareness or if you are striving too hard for results. Remember that trying too hard to increase hand or foot warmth has the opposite effect of bringing about cooling.

If a cooling trend persists, change the goal of your session to hand cooling. In self-regulation training, learning two-way control of a physiological function such as body peripheral temperature is indicative of increased mastery of the technique. If you unexpectedly find yourself experiencing a cooling trend, take advantage of this by seeing how cool you can make your hands and feet. You can learn just as much from cooling as you can from warming.

CHAPTER · 8

The Link Between Breathing and Blood Pressure: Three-Part Complete Breathing

Of the techniques we learned, deep breathing was the most beneficial to me. I never realized that hypertensives didn't know how to breathe. One would think that it's a very natural act; . . . in fact, breathing was the hardest for me to learn, but I think the most useful. I keep it in mind and quite often still catch myself . . . breathing the wrong way. Then I get into the practice, and it has an instantaneous effect of making my hand temperature go up.

—RICHARD
Tax attorney
HART participant

If you would foster a calm spirit, first regulate your breathing; for when that is under control, the heart will lie at peace; but when breathing is spasmodic, then it will be troubled. Therefore, before attempting anything, first regulate your breathing on which your temper will be softened, your spirit calmed.

—KARIBA EKKEN
(seventeenth century)

NOT LONG AGO, after the sudden death of her husband, Ann's blood pressure skyrocketed. For months, her hypertension remained in poor control, despite the multiple medications prescribed by her physician. Both she and her son (a doctor) were very concerned, so Ann decided to try the HART Program techniques.

Within just a few sessions, Ann significantly reduced her blood pressure. Autogenic training, relaxation, and breathing exercises brought her blood pressure down to almost normal.

Ann experienced a major breakthrough when she incorporated the breathing techniques you will learn in this chapter. Following her first training session in this Three-Part Complete Breathing process, she began to get readings below 140/90 at home. That week, her blood pressure was measured in her doctor's office—and for the first time, it was back under control at 130/80. Her blood pressure had declined and had stayed low even though she had had a severe asthma attack the night before. With the calming effect of the Three-Part Complete Breathing process, she was able to overcome the sense of fear and panic that her asthma attacks usually evoked. Ann said, "It is a real triumph."

By increasing your awareness of how you breathe, and incorporating this chapter's breathing techniques into your relaxation practice, you will have a powerful tool capable of quieting your thoughts, calming your emotions, deepening your relaxation, and regaining control of your blood pressure.

How is this possible? Most simply, like blood pressure, your breathing is under the control of your autonomic or involuntary nervous system. However, unlike blood pressure, breathing **can** be consciously and directly controlled. By altering your patterns of breathing, you can gain access to and directly influence your autonomic system in the direction of greater relaxation, while interrupting the physiological arousal that can lead to high blood pressure and stress-related disorders. Since you take about 21,000 breaths a day, you therefore have countless opportunities to influence your autonomic balance—and thus your blood pressure.

While it is possible to go for weeks without food and days without water, even a few minutes without breathing can undermine your most vital life functions. No wonder learning and practicing the Three-Part Complete Breathing process is an essential part of your self-regulatory program. If you want to normalize your hypertension, this breathing technique can be one of your most important allies.

As Richard, a tax attorney who successfully normalized his blood pressure, recounted, "Breathing was the most important skill I learned . . . . My wife knew how to breathe because she sings in a choir; my minister knew how to breathe because he preaches. But I had never learned how to breathe correctly until I began practicing the breathing techniques in this program—and what a difference it has made!"

WHAT HAPPENS WHEN YOU BREATHE

How often do you give any thought to your breathing? Probably rarely. Yet thousands of times a day, this essential, life-sustaining process takes place. With each quiet and relaxed breath, you inhale and exhale about one pint of air. However, by breathing more deeply and fully, using the techniques in this chapter, you can easily increase this to seven or eight pints of air, utilizing much more of your natural lung capacity. The oxygen that you draw in is critical for the proper functioning of all your cells and tissues. Breath is life.

The breathing process begins with air being brought in through the nose, where it is warmed and moistened by the mucous membranes as it makes its way into the body. The air then travels down the windpipe—a channel about four inches long and less than an inch in diameter. This windpipe divides into two primary bronchi, one directed into each lung. In turn, these bronchi branch into many smaller air passages called bronchioles. At the end of these bronchioles are the alveoli, which are tiny air sacs that line the lungs like ripe, full clusters of grapes. There are a staggering 300 million of these alveoli in each lung.

The diaphragm is the primary muscle that keeps the breathing process going. It is a dome-shaped muscle that separates the abdomen from the chest, and with each inhalation, as the ribs move upward and outward, the diaphragm moves downward. This expands the space in the chest and allows oxygen-rich air from the outside to be drawn into the lungs. Oxygen then makes its way into the bloodstream and circulates to every part of the body, replenishing and nourishing every cell.

When you exhale, your diaphragm recoils and relaxes. It pushes up toward the chest, emptying the lungs of carbon dioxide that has been carried there from the body's tissues.

The speed and depth of breathing are controlled by the brain—specifically, a group of cells at the base of the brain in the so-called "respiratory center." The brain senses when there is too much carbon dioxide in the blood, at which time it communicates with the muscles involved in breathing, and orders the respiration to accelerate. This provides the cells with the oxygen they need to expel the carbon dioxide that has built up within them.

For breathing to function properly, everything has to work efficiently and in sync: the brain and nervous system that control the entire operation; the lungs that work like bellows; and the diaphragm and rib cage, which are like the driving motor. At the same time, the heart pumps, and the arteries, veins, and capillaries carry oxygen and remove carbon dioxide throughout the body. It is a complex and beautifully-efficient process.

BREATHING, BLOOD PRESSURE, AND HEALTH

Breathing patterns are closely associated with your mental and emotional state as well as your physical health. Observe your breath during your daily life. Note how it changes with different psychological states.

When you are calm and relaxed, it probably becomes deeper and more rhythmic. When you are feeling stressed, it is probably choppier and more shallow. When you are startled or afraid—part of the alarm or fight-or-flight response—you may find yourself holding your breath.

For hypertensive patients, breathing patterns often play at least some role in their illness. Clinical observations at the Menninger Foundation—and at other centers where biobehavioral techniques are used—indicate that persons with high blood pressure and other cardiovascular illnesses generally have breathing practices that are counterproductive to good health. They are often "reverse breathers," which means they expand their chest before their abdomen when inhaling. Or they may have arrhythmic, gasping, or breath-holding patterns.

All these breathing irregularities can be associated with hypertension. They are the antithesis of the even, natural breathing patterns that most of us had as infants. Babies instinctively breathe abdominally or diaphragmatically. However, between infancy and adulthood, without even realizing it, many people somehow lose their naturally perfect breathing patterns. Fortunately, however, they can be regained.

Poor posture, extra pounds, lack of regular aerobic exercise, and our response to the stresses and challenges of life can all adversely impact our breathing. So can smoking, which literally sears and explodes the delicate air sacs in our lungs that receive oxygen. Aging itself can erode the functioning of our respiratory system; over the years, the air cells in our lungs can contract in size and let in less oxygen, causing a decrease in vital capacity.

Let's pause a moment to define a term. *Vital capacity* is the scientific term for the amount of air that we can exhale slowly after maximum inhalation. It represents our greatest possible breathing capacity.

Few people know that vital capacity is one of the most important predictors of longevity. Many experts believe that establishing healthy breathing patterns, exercising regularly, and abstaining from smoking can postpone and even prevent deterioration of our vital capacity, helping to keep air cells at their normal size, and maintaining and even reclaiming a fuller lung capacity. In essence, cultivating better breathing patterns—together with other healthy lifestyle habits—may retard the aging process and assist you in maintaining a fuller breathing capacity throughout your life.

HART patients have discovered that not only can the practice of breathing calm their mind and deepen their relaxation, it can also assist in reducing their anxiety, depression, and irritability. In addition, since the body's energy needs are provided by oxygen plus glucose, breathing more deeply and fully can provide considerably more energy, while improving concentration and combating fatigue.

In this chapter, you'll learn how to modify your less-than-optimal breathing habits and adopt a healthier pattern by changing the rate, depth, and quality of your breathing.

THE YOGIC INFLUENCE

Much of what we know about breathing techniques comes from the yogic tradition, a two thousand year old methodology for developing and unifying body, mind, and spirit leading to full self-realization (the oneness of self with creation). For many thousands of years, yogis, practitioners of yoga, recognized the relationship between our consciousness, health, and breath, maintaining that our very life force is carried in our breath. As a result, they developed a science of breathing control called *pranayama*. The root word *prana* means not only breath, air, energy, and strength, but life itself. The second half of the word, *ayama*, means expansion or extending. The yogis liken breathing to the "string that controls the kite"—the kite being analogous to the mind. When breathing is unsteady or haphazard, the mind vacillates; but when breathing is gently brought back into a rhythmic pattern, the mind and emotions become steady, clear, and balanced.

The link between breath, mind, emotions, and health is expressed throughout our language. A strong emotion can "take our breath away." When exhausted, we may be "ready to expire;" when we're ready to go forward, we call it "getting a second wind." We count on "inspiration" for our best ideas and to energize us.

Psychologists and physicians are now discovering that proper breathing offers a powerful way of quieting the nervous system and bringing greater emotional equilibrium and health, as well as making the respiratory system more robust and enhancing vital capacity. Sages and saints from every major tradition have recognized that rhythmic, deep, balanced breathing can bring a sense of peace and joyfulness to one's life. Many also believe it may extend the life span and thus they measure a person's life not by years, but by the number of breaths. To promote longevity, the yogis suggest thinking of extending and deepening the breathing process as drawing breath all the way down to one's abdomen or even heels; the longer, slower, and deeper the breath, the longer the life.

BECOMING AWARE OF YOUR OWN BREATHING PATTERNS

Are you aware of your own breathing patterns? Do you breathe from your abdomen and diaphragm, or are you a chest or thoracic breather? For the next few minutes, pay attention to your breathing without attempting to change it in any way. To begin, place one hand on your abdomen, just below the rib cage, and the other hand on your chest. Observe your hands as you breathe. Where does the movement begin and end when you inhale and exhale? Where does most of the movement occur; lower abdomen, upper abdomen, chest, or all three?

If the hand over your abdomen moves downward or not at all and the hand on your chest rises, you are breathing from the thorax or with your chest; you are a "reverse breather." However, if the hand over your abdomen moves upward as you inhale, you are breathing from the abdomen or diaphragm.

As we've been discussing, it is much healthier to breathe diaphragmatically (from the diaphragm). In this type of breathing pattern, considerably more oxygen is drawn into your lower lungs. The lower lungs have considerably more ability to absorb oxygen than the upper lungs. By contrast, in thoracic breathing, air stays high in your chest, and your lungs don't fill as adequately as they should; in fact, you use only about one-fourth of your lung capacity when you breathe from your thorax. As a result, your heart has to work harder, pumping more blood to transport the same amount of oxygen.

There are other advantages to diaphragmatic breathing. It does a better job of pushing waste products such as carbon dioxide out of the lungs. Thoracic breathers inhale and exhale shallowly, so much more residual carbon dioxide remains in their lungs, which can contribute to anxiety and exhaustion. Also, as the diaphragm itself contracts and relaxes during breathing, this action gently massages the internal organs, stimulating circulation and helping internal organs to function better.

If you breathe thoracically (from the thorax, or primarily from the upper chest) it is time to change. You may need to go through an "unlearning" process to shift to diaphragmatic breathing. Fortunately, even habits you've developed over many years can be modified. For instance, if you learned to stand up straight, with your chest out and your stomach held tightly in, breathing from the diaphragm can be quite difficult. You may need to soften your abdomen and allow it to move as you shift from thoracic to diaphragmatic breathing. Similarly, if you tend to sit or stand with your chest collapsed and concaved, this can also impede diaphragmatic breathing. You may need to open and expand your chest by lengthening the space between your breastbone and navel through lifting upward from the breastbone, thus enabling you to use more of your lung capacity. Take a moment to open and expand your chest and feel the difference in your ability to breathe.

Once you start and become accustomed to breathing from the diaphragm—the preferable way for lowering blood pressure—you will experience a refreshing, tranquil feeling of relaxation. This is the type of instant reinforcement that will encourage you to begin each of your daily relaxation sessions with a few minutes of the Three-Part Complete Breathing technique. Later, when you begin the stress management phase of the program, your familiarity with this technique and its impact will motivate you to incorporate healthier diaphragmatic breathing patterns into your daily life.

THREE-PART COMPLETE BREATHING: THE WAY TO BREATHE FOR LOWER BLOOD PRESSURE

The Three-Part Complete Breathing process consists of deep, gentle inhaling and exhaling at a constant rate—smoothly, without strain, and without pausing at the top or the bottom of your breathing cycle. Sometimes this breath pattern is referred to as "triangular breathing;" if you were to monitor it on a respiration gauge, it would make a triangular record on a polygraph strip. This pattern of breathing allows you to inhale about seven times as much air as shallow or thoracic breathing. That means a greater supply of oxygen for use by your brain and body. Also, increasing the volume of the air you breathe will slow your rate of respiration and decelerate your heart rate.

The Three-Part Complete Breathing technique is a continuous, sequential process in which the lungs progressively fill from bottom to top with oxygen as you inhale, and then empty from top to bottom as you exhale. It is analogous to filling and emptying a glass of water: First, the lower portion of the glass fills, then the middle and upper portions. When pouring water from the glass, the water flows first from the top, then the middle, and finally the bottom.

In a similar way, the lower lungs fill up first, as your diaphragm moves downward and air is drawn into the vacuum created in the chest cavity. Then the middle lungs fill, and finally the uppermost portion, as the lungs become completely filled. During exhaling, the air first flows out of the upper, then the middle, and finally the lower parts of the lungs.

LEARNING THREE-PART COMPLETE BREATHING X

The Three-Part Complete Breathing process is a straightforward technique to learn, and you will begin to enjoy its benefits immediately. Once you learn the basic technique described in the three steps below, start each relaxation session with a few minutes of this breathing. You may wish to do a few practice sessions using a mirror to check your technique. With practice a rapid look at your torso and your inner awareness will let you know how you are breathing.

1. **Establishing the Basic Pattern of Three-Part Complete Breathing.** Start by sitting comfortably and symmetrically, with your chest open, your back straight yet relaxed, your legs apart, and your feet flat on the floor. Throughout this exercise, both inhalations and exhalations are done through your nostrils. Until you have learned the proper inward movement of your abdomen as you exhale, place your hands over your abdomen. Gently but firmly, press your abdomen inward as you exhale completely. Then, as you inhale, allow your abdomen to expand, followed by the expansion of your chest and torso. At the crest of the inhalation, your collarbone will rise slightly. As you exhale, let your chest and then your abdomen descend in a wave. Exhale completely. Then slowly inhale again. This is the basic pattern of the Three-Part Complete Breathing process. Establish this pattern, then proceed to step 2.

2. **Smoothing Out Your Breathing.** As you continue to practice the basic pattern of the Three-Part Complete Breathing process, watch your abdomen and torso. Make your breathing long, deep, and continuous, without pausing between inhaling and exhaling. Smooth out any stops, starts, or abrupt motions. These are subtle adjustments; observe your breathing carefully and make any necessary alterations that allow your breath to be smooth and continuous. When you are comfortable with this pattern, go on to step 3.

3. **Extending and Equalizing the Length of Your Breath.** As you continue the Three-Part Complete Breathing process, inhale to a count of four or five for each "in" breath, and exhale to a count of four or five for each "out" breath—or use whatever count is comfortable for you. Count the length of your inhalations and exhalations and adjust them so they are of equal duration.

   In the ensuing days and weeks of practice, increase the length of the cycles, gradually and without strain. Over time, extend each breath to a count of eight to ten as you inhale, and an equal length as you exhale. Practice the Three-Part Complete Breathing process comfortably, and gradually expand the depth and duration of your breath.

MAXIMIZING THE EFFECTIVENESS OF THE TECHNIQUE

After becoming acquainted with the basics of the Three-Part Complete Breathing process, you can further develop your mastery of this technique by practicing a more refined version of what you've already learned. You can pre-record the comprehensive Three-Part Complete Breathing text that follows on a cassette tape: read it slowly, allow ample time to follow each instruction, then play it back as you proceed through the exercise. Or you may decide to read the instructions as you do the technique, giving yourself plenty of time to follow along.

As with autogenic training, be sure to take some baseline measurements both before you start the more refined Three-Part Complete Breathing technique, and after you finish the session. This will tell you immediately how the process affects your vital signs. Find a comfortable chair, put your monitoring equipment within easy reach, then measure your blood pressure, pulse rate, and finger or toe temperature, and enter the readings on your data sheet. Remember to take the same readings after you finish your practice. Also, make sure you have cushions or towel rolls available to increase your comfort, soften the diaphragm, release tension, and allow breathing to begin low in the abdominal region and become effortlessly deep.

BEGIN YOUR SESSIONS WITH A RECLINING OR STANDING STRETCH

It's best to begin with either a brief reclining or standing stretch to open the chest and breathing and release residual muscular tension.

Reclining Stretch. Lie down on your back on a comfortable but firm surface with your arms resting on the ground, extended over your head. Close your eyes and imagine that your body is as pliable as elastic.

Start the stretch in the hip region, and feel your body extending in both directions. Imagine being held by your wrists and ankles and being stretched fully. Stretch downward sequentially through your hips . . . thighs . . . calves . . . ankles. . . and toes. At the same time, stretch upward through your abdomen . . . your back . . . chest . . . shoulders . . . neck . . . head . . . arms . . . wrists . . . hands . . . fingers. Keep breathing while you stretch.

Now, scan your body, looking for any areas you might stretch even more. Feel that additional extension taking place. Elongate your body even further by stretching your legs, calves, and feet as much as possible in one direction, and your torso, arms, and hands in the other. Hold this full stretch 10 to 20 seconds and then continue breathing.

Next, relax completely and breathe deeply. Repeat this stretch-relax-breathe cycle two more times.

Standing Stretch. Begin by standing with your feet apart about the distance of your hips. Raise your arms above your head, reaching toward the ceiling. As you inhale, begin your stretch from your ankles, and gradually feel each part of your body stretching upward. Feel the upward extension moving from your feet and ankles up through your calves . . . legs . . . thighs . . . torso . . . neck . . . head . . . arms . . . hands . . . to the tips of your fingers, until you are maximally elongated.

Reach upward and continue to breathe as you elongate. Stretch as completely as you can while reaching upward.

To increase your extension even further, you may wish to imagine reaching up past the ceiling, through the sky and toward the stars.

Then relax, exhaling completely. Breathe.

Now that you have stretched, be aware of differences in how you're breathing. Chances are you can breathe more easily and deeply. Repeat this stretch-breathe-relax cycle three times before getting into a comfortable position for relaxing.

THREE-PART COMPLETE BREATHING: REFINING THE PROCESS

Now that you've opened and deepened your breathing through stretching, you are ready to further refine your Three-Part Complete Breathing technique. If you are lying down, and you choose to use cushions or bolsters under your head and back, now is the time to put them in place.

1. With your eyes closed, relax your facial muscles, the muscles around the eyes and the eyes themselves. This will help calm your mind. Relax your inner ears . . . Listen receptively to the quiet, smooth, soundless resonance of your breathing . . . Your breath need never be rough, loud or uneven . . . Your ears will provide exquisitely sensitive feedback suggesting when to adjust the quality of your breath.
2. Exhale the air from your lungs as fully as possible, comfortably and without strain. This expels the stale, residual air from your lower lungs and makes more room for fresh, oxygenated life-giving breath to flow in during your next inhalation.
3. Inhale through both nostrils . . . slowly . . . steadily . . . smoothly . . . deeply . . . completely. As you inhale, feel your abdomen and then your chest expand in a smooth, continuous, wave-like motion as your breath flows into your lower, middle and upper lungs.
4. Without pausing, exhale through both nostrils . . . slowly . . . steadily . . . evenly . . . smoothly . . . deeply . . . completely . . . As

you exhale, feel your abdominal muscles move in toward your spine, pressing out the residual air in your lower lungs. Initially, accentuate this movement by placing both hands on your abdomen and gently but firmly pressing your abdomen inward to help you exhale completely.

5. Without pausing, inhale. Feel the breath flowing through your nostrils and into your lungs . . . slowly . . . evenly . . . steadily . . . smoothly . . . deeply . . . completely.

6. For the next few minutes count the length of your "in" breaths and "out" breaths. Make them of equal duration. Begin with a count of four or five for each. Gradually and gently over time, extend the length of your inhalations and exhalations until you can comfortably and without strain expand your "in" breaths and "out" breaths to a count of ten each.

7. Continue this cycle of slow, smooth, complete inhalations and exhalations. Consciously observe and feel the flow of your breath. Allow your breathing to be even and continuous without pauses, stops, or starts. Note and correct any jerkiness, unevenness or roughness in your breathing. Listen to your breath- . . . breathe steadily and without sound.

As you inhale, imagine your breath flowing in a wave from your heels all the way to your head, filling you with renewed vitality. As you exhale, allow your breath to flow out again in a smooth wave into the greater ocean of air around you—and relax, completely and deeply. You may begin to feel a sense of tingling or warmth.

As you inhale, let your breath flow in a wave all the way through your body, from your toes to your head.

On your exhalation, as your breath flows out in a wave, feel the vitality of your breath being absorbed by your body . . . and your relaxation deepening . . . Allow yourself to enjoy the pleasurable sense of calm and inward quiet.

8. At this point, you may bring the session to a close—or if you wish, continue your self-regulation session, perhaps by using whatever autogenic phrases work best for your hand and foot warming and relaxation practice.

When you are ready to end the session, inhale and take a long, complete stretch. Then, feeling deeply relaxed, refreshed, and ready to bring a greater sense of balance and clarity to the rest of your day or evening, open your eyes. Finish by taking and recording your blood pressure, pulse, and hand or foot temperature. Take a few moments to reflect on the refinements you want to incorporate into your ongoing practice.

OPTIMIZING THE BENEFITS OF THREE-PART COMPLETE BREATHING

Here are a few suggestions to keep in mind during your practice. First, be sure to begin the breathing portion of the session by exhaling completely in order to expel the stale, deoxygenated air.

If you are having difficulty opening or lengthening your breath, pay particular attention to your posture. Make whatever adjustments are needed so your chest is open and unconstricted. Make sure your clothing, belts, and other accessories are comfortable and do not constrict your breathing.

For the next week, concentrate on refining the Three-Part Complete Breathing technique, and practice it for three to five minutes at the start of each relaxation session, then use the autogenic phrases that work best for warming your hands and feet. Remember to take and record your blood pressure, pulse, and hand or foot temperature before and after each session.

Periodically, review the following ten pointers for effective breathing.

TEN POINTERS FOR EFFECTIVE THREE-PART COMPLETE BREATHING PRACTICE ⎯⎯⎯⎯⎯⎯⎯⎯⎯⎯⎯⎯⎯⎯

1. Begin each relaxation session with a few minutes of Three-Part Complete Breathing.
2. Before you start, stretch to make breathing easier. While either reclining or sitting, repeat the stretch-relax-breathe cycle three times.
3. Adjust your posture so your chest is open rather than compressed. Use pillows or bolsters under your head and back if you find it more comfortable or if your breathing feels tight.
4. Loosen any clothing, ties, belts, or accessories that might constrict your breathing.
5. Begin your breathing practice by exhaling completely to expel any residual, stale air. Breathe through your nose rather than your mouth.
6. Breathe from your diaphragm—that is, more abdominally—rather than from your thorax or solely with your chest.
7. Make your inhalations and exhalations of equal duration. Gradually, extend the duration of your breaths until you can comfortably inhale to a count of ten, then exhale to a count of ten.
8. Periodically observe your torso as you breathe to make sure the movement is smooth, wavelike, and continuous without jerks,

or stops and starts. Listen to make sure you are breathing quietly.

9. If your mind wanders or you become distracted during your practice, rather than reacting, criticizing, or judging yourself, merely be aware when this occurs and immediately redirect your attention back to your breathing techniques.

10. Stay within your comfort zone. Stop if you feel strain or dizziness. Your practice is meant to bring about a sense of inner quiet, relaxation, joy, and ease.

In the next chapter, you can use the Three-Part Complete Breathing process as a lead-in to Systematic Muscular Relaxation. In the meantime, you will find that breathing practice has its own intrinsic rewards. The Three-Part Complete Breathing process is one of the most powerful methods of quieting your autonomic nervous system and deepening your relaxation. Along with the other self-regulatory techniques that are part of the HART Program, this breathing process will help you achieve your goal of lowering your blood pressure.

CHAPTER · 9

Systematic Muscular Relaxation

If you relax your skeletal muscles sufficiently [those over which you have control], the internal muscles [including the heart, blood vessels and colon] tend to relax likewise.

—EDMUND JACOBSON, M.D.
You Must Relax

. . . [I]n most kinds of anxiety the physical expression of anxiety, if not a good share of the anxiety itself, is the unfelt, unseen muscle tension that braces the body against fearful situations without consciousness being much aware that tension exists, generally not until long after the cause for anxiety has been removed.

—DR. BARBARA BROWN
*Stress and the Art of
Biofeedback*

IN OUR CULTURE, there has been a tendency to overlook the role that muscles can play in the health and illness of body and mind. However, if we take a close look, we can see that the human body is predominantly muscle. Each of us has more than 600 muscles and they are essential to every movement we make, from walking up a flight of stairs to the smallest nuance in facial expression. Muscles enable our hearts to beat, our pupils to contract and expand, our arteries to constrict and dilate, and food to move through our digestive system. They enable us to express our love or fear and to work and play in the world around us. Indeed, we cannot make a move without our muscles.

Since muscles are so essential to our well-being, you may not be surprised to learn that they can also play a key role in the onset—as well as in the recovery from—stress-related disorders. There is, in fact, a three-quarters-of-a-century history in the West of muscular relaxation-based treatment of disorders ranging from anxiety and ulcers to cardiac arrhythmias and hypertension.

This chapter will introduce you to the technique called Systematic Muscular Relaxation. Like autogenics, it can help raise your body's peripheral temperature to levels indicative of deep relaxation, while also reducing pulse rate, decreasing blood pressure, and giving you access to a deep, enjoyable sense of mental, emotional, and physical ease.

WHAT CAUSES MUSCULAR TENSION?

Our bodies have two major types of muscles: *striate muscles*, involved in movements under our voluntary control; and *smooth muscles*, found in the internal organs, including the heart and blood vessels, which are predominantly controlled by the Autonomic Nervous System (ANS). Research shows that by deeply relaxing the striate muscles over which we have control, we can actually expand this relaxation to include the muscles of the heart and blood vessels.

Our muscles, which exist in pairs, are superbly designed for movement. For movement to take place, some muscles must contract while others relax. Tension occurs when muscles tighten without any body movement; this is a common reaction of our bodies to stress. Muscle tension is literally a shortness or contracting of muscle fibers, while relaxation—the opposite of tension—is a state of rest or an absence of effort.

Increases in muscle tension—like rises in heart rate and blood pressure—are part of the body's automatic alarm reaction. Muscles tense as the body mobilizes to fight, freeze, or flee in response to a perceived threat to our social or physical well-being. Most individuals respond to social pressures with increased muscle tension called "bracing," which Dr. Barbara Brown has described as "the muscles' act of preparing to defend or freeze or to avoid unpleasantness by having the important action muscles ready to move or stand by."

The muscular tension you feel from knotted shoulders, an aching back, a tight jaw, or a stiff neck is one of your body's ways of letting you know you are under stress. Many times, the body tenses in response to stress **before** it is recognized by the conscious mind; this increase in muscle tension can go undetected even while it continues to increase, eroding your physical and psychological well-being.

Over time, muscle tightness and tension, which many of us carry in our neck, back, shoulders, and forehead, can take its toll. Initially, tight muscles contribute to irritability, anxiety, fatigue, and susceptibility to minor conditions like colds and the flu. Over the long term, muscular tension plays a role in the onset of stress-related disorders like high blood pressure, cardiovascular disease, arthritis, and ulcers.

By learning to detect and release tension in your muscles through Systematic Muscular Relaxation, you will master an additional, important self-regulatory skill that can assist you in achieving your blood pressure reduction goals.

THE NEED TO RELAX

Many individuals are faced with frequent if not almost continuous stress, whether from the small, cumulative hassles and demands of everyday life or from major life changes. For example, people who work in sales must deal cordially with customers and employees, no matter how harassed they may feel. Stress is felt by the small entrepreneur trying to keep a business afloat, the householder attempting to keep grocery spending within the family budget, the supervisor in middle management who is accountable for meeting increasing performance objectives, the factory worker who must perform repetitive tasks every day, and the individual faced with family dissonance, illness or the loss of a significant other, or the strain of making time for both work and family.

Without an effective way to unwind and restore themselves, the body and mind literally begin to tighten up and, correspondingly, resilience and resistance to illness wears down. Unless we manage our stress in constructive ways, such as with relaxation techniques and healthy lifestyle habits, there is a tendency to look for relief from stress by reaching for a drink, tranquilizer, social drug, cigarette, or junk food—methods of coping that can themselves be health risks.

You may also not realize that you are under stress. Because your consciousness is selective at any given time, you are probably only aware of a portion of what is going on around and within you. For example, as you're reading, unless you take a moment to redirect part of your awareness to your body, you may not be aware of the seat or the surface beneath you, or of the degree of tightness or relaxation around your eyes, facial muscles, shoulders, arms, or back.

Yet by even briefly redirecting your attention to how your body is feeling, you may discover areas of tightness that you can then take steps to improve. Relaxing your muscles is a two-part process: First, you become aware of any tightness or tension, then you intentionally allow that part of you to release and relax.

Some patients are surprised to find out that their bodies have been holding hidden tension. This was Edward's experience: "I don't think I ever really noticed how tense I tended to be. But just going through the exercises, I suddenly found that my shoulders were stiff, my neck was stiff, and I immediately took some steps to relieve this tension."

RELEASING MUSCLE TENSION

How is it possible that muscle tension can build to the point where it contributes to psychological and physical disorders? A number of factors may come into play. The stresses of life are common if not continuous for many individuals. Although some spontaneous relaxation occurs after tension rises, this relaxation takes place slowly. Often, tension levels are still high when yet another stressful event occurs, increasing the tension even further.

Dr. Barbara Brown has observed, "If muscles are not given relief from tension by relaxation or a change in activity, the muscle fibers physiologically 'adapt' to the increased states of tension. It is as if there were some deficiency in the internal regulating systems. When it comes to sensing how long muscle fibers have been tense, the system seems to become inefficient (as if we were not designed to handle so much social stress)."

Sensors within the muscles themselves relay messages of tension to the muscle-control areas in the brain. Unless the muscle tightness becomes severe, however, our attention is most often occupied with the stressful situation itself. There may be little or no awareness of the increasing tightness in the body.

Dr. Brown and other researchers have hypothesized that active cortical processes may actually block or inhibit our awareness of muscle tension; this has the effect of keeping the muscles on alert, ready for action. These muscles will tend to maintain their tension levels until the stressful situation is resolved or recognized, and emotional adjustments are made.

In effect, a circular feedback loop exists between our mind and muscles. By mentally rehashing or constantly ruminating about irritating or stressful situations, we can dramatically increase muscle tension. This muscular tension itself can then significantly elevate emotional tension and stressful thoughts, which in turn further raises muscle tension. In this interactive cycle, a stressed mind contributes to tense muscles. (If you have doubts about the existence of this cycle, see and feel what happens to your muscles and mind if you think about a stressful event over and over.)

Through the practice of relaxation techniques, muscle tension is released, and in turn, so is the alerting effect upon the brain that can interfere with relaxation. As this occurs, muscles are able to more easily release and resume normal functioning, and emotional tension subsides. During moments of complete relaxation, few if any muscle fibers are active; as a result, you'll feel calm and alert, and your muscles will be at ease. Systematic Muscular Relaxation intervenes by directing your thoughts to the present by concentrating all your attention on the muscle groups that you are progressively relaxing. With your thoughts focused on the moment, your mind is drawn away from dwelling on the events and people contributing to the stress and anxiety in your life. This helps relieve the tension in your muscles and ultimately contributes to a decrease in your blood pressure. In effect, you are blocking the mental processes and muscular tightness that create stress and activate increases in your blood pressure.

Systematic Muscular Relaxation goes to the root of the stress cycle, directly affecting the muscle fibers themselves. As was mentioned earlier in this chapter, muscles can perform either of two functions—contracting or relaxing—depending on the instructions they receive from a control system in the brain. These messages are communicated in just a fraction of a second through an intricate neural system, by nerve impulses that either stimulate the muscle fibers to contract, or interfere with that directive and thus allow them to relax. Even though we often think of the muscles as independent entities that we can train and exercise, it is the **brain** that regulates all their activity. The muscles and their tiny fibers need the brain's continuous cooperation. Just as we can do nothing without our muscles, our muscles can do nothing without directives from the brain and central nervous system.

MUSCULAR RELAXATION AND TREATMENT OF ILLNESS

The pioneering work of Dr. Edmund Jacobson at Harvard, Cornell, and the University of Chicago has provided us with much of what we know about the therapeutic benefits of muscular relaxation. Dr. Jacobson researched the benefits of a systematic approach to relaxing the musculature, and how it could help treat a wide range of disorders, including hypertension, cardiac arrhythmias, coronary heart disease, anxiety, ulcers, and chronic pain.

Dr. Jacobson discovered that when individuals successfully learned muscular relaxation, they could relax not only the striate muscles, which are under voluntary control, but also the smooth muscles that were once thought to be beyond conscious control—including those in the cardiovascular system and the gastrointestinal tract.

In this research, Dr. Jacobson also extensively examined the interconnectedness between muscle tension, illness, and anxiety. He hypothesized that if people could reduce the tension in their muscles, they could also relieve their anxiety and stress, and more effectively recover from stress-related illness. His primary thesis—and one of his foremost contributions to the field of psychosomatic medicine—is that anxiety and relaxation are mutually exclusive. He wrote that "an anxious mind cannot exist within a relaxed body."

GETTING STARTED WITH SYSTEMATIC MUSCULAR RELAXATION

Essentially, Systematic Muscular Relaxation (SMR) involves focusing your attention on each part of your body in turn, beginning with your feet and moving to your head. In this way, you become fully aware of the sensations in each part of your body, and can suggest that each part of your body relax completely and deeply.

By using thermal feedback, you will be able to see how Systematic Muscular Relaxation affects your hand or foot temperature. As you recall, muscles in the arterial walls contract and then widen in response to sympathetic nervous system activity. Many HART patients observe that as they release areas of subtle yet chronically-held tension—for example, around their eyes, jaw, neck, and shoulders—they see a definite increase in body peripheral temperature. Pay special attention to discovering those areas where you hold chronic tension and relaxing them as you proceed through your SMR sequence.

As with autogenic training, you may either tape the SMR text in this chapter with your tape recorder and then play back the tape as you actually practice the technique; or read through the exercise as you practice it, following the instructions as you move along. Remember to use a pleasant, relaxed voice and pace that will encourage relaxation.

During your first week of practice, proceed through SMR more slowly as you move from one bodily region to the next, giving yourself time to scan for any tightness and allowing your sense of relaxation to deepen. Repeat each instruction twice, and feel how your muscles relax and release even more. With time, your muscles will be able to relax much more rapidly yet just as completely.

Some people use a tape recorder during only one of their daily sessions, proceeding through the exercise unassisted during the other. The technique soon becomes second nature, and they no longer need to rely on the tape.

Remember, for at least one relaxation session per day, begin by taking your blood pressure, pulse, and hand temperature. Jot down the readings on your data sheet. Rate the level of tension or relaxation you're feeling on a −10 to +10 point scale; give yourself a rating of −10 if you're feeling extremely tense, +10 if you're completely relaxed, or a number somewhere in between.

After you can warm your hands to 95.5–96 degrees (the criteria for deep relaxation), be sure to shift your thermistor placement to your feet and practice warming them to 90–93 degrees.

The final technique in the sequence—imagery—is the focus of the next chapter.

PRACTICING SYSTEMATIC MUSCULAR RELAXATION

1. Briefly stretch using the stretch-relax-breathe sequence.
2. Settle into a comfortable position, and focus your attention on your breathing.

    For the next few minutes, deepen and extend your breath with the Three-Part Complete Breathing technique.
3. Begin Systematic Muscular Relaxation by focusing your attention on your toes, feet and ankles. Be aware of how relaxed or tense they are. Inwardly suggest that they relax . . . "My toes . . . feet . . . and ankles . . . relax." Allow them to relax. "My toes . . . feet . . . and ankles . . . relax." Feel the relaxation deepening.
4. Feel your awareness flow upward into your calves and knees. "My calves and knees, relax . . . My calves and knees, relax."
5. Let your awareness float upward into your thighs. "My thighs, relax" . . . Feel the relaxation deepening . . . "My thighs, relax."
6. Let your awareness flow into your stomach and pelvic region. Be aware of any tightness or tension. Now inwardly suggest, "My stomach and pelvic region, relax" . . . Feel your stomach and pelvic muscles softening, relaxing, letting go, and relaxing more deeply. "My stomach and pelvic region, relax" . . . Continue long, deep, and complete abdominal breaths. Feel your relaxation deepening with each exhalation.
7. Let your awareness flow into your buttocks. "My buttocks, relax . . . My buttocks, relax." Feel your buttocks become heavier and yield to gravity.
8. Let your awareness flow upward into your lower, middle and upper back. Be aware of any tightness or tension. Inwardly suggest, "My lower back, mid-back, and upper back, relax" . . . Feel the muscles of your back relaxing and letting go . . . "My lower back, my mid-back, my upper back, relax." Let the relaxation deepen with each exhalation.
9. Let your awareness flow into your chest region. Be aware of any tightness. "My chest, relax" . . . Feel your chest softening, relaxing and releasing . . . "My chest, relax."
10. Bring your awareness to your shoulders. Be aware of any tension or tightness. Allow your shoulders to release and relax . . . "My shoulders, relax." If you wish, gently tighten your shoulders, pull them up toward your ears, then allow them to release and relax downward . . . "My shoulders, relax." Allow any residual tightness to flow out with your exhalation.

11. In the same way, bring your attention to each successive body part. As you do, be aware of any tightness or tension, then allow that part of you to relax. Feel the relaxation deepening as your muscles release and relax. Repeating your relaxation phrases twice to deepen this process.

    As you move from one part of your body to the next, allow enough time for that region of your body to relax as completely as possible.

    "My hands, wrists, lower arms, elbows and upper arms, relax" . . .

    "My neck, relax" . . .

    "My head, relax" . . . Allow your head to roll gently from side to side. Feel the relaxation deepening.

    "My jaw, relax"

    "My lips and tongue, relax" . . .

    "My forehead, relax" . . .

    "My eyes, relax" . . .

    "My ears, relax" . . .

    "My brain, relax" . . .

    "My lungs, relax" . . .

    "My heart, relax" . . .

    "My entire body and mind are completely and deeply relaxed" . . .

    "With each exhalation, I am allowing my body to relax even deeper" . . .

    With practice, you will be able to merely focus your awareness on successive body parts, intend that they relax, and feel the relaxation occurring.

12. Now, take a few moments to gently scan your body, moving your awareness in a wave from your head to your feet, releasing any residual tightness or tension that may remain and feeling your sense of relaxation deepening even more. At the close of this sequential relaxation process, say to yourself, "My entire body and mind are completely and deeply relaxed." Take a few moments to enjoy this experience. Allow the pleasant sense of relaxation, inner quiet, and ease to persist as you either bring the session to a close, or continue it with the practice of the autogenic phrases and images that have been most effective for relaxation and warming your hands and feet.

REFLECTING ON YOUR EXPERIENCE

When you've finished your session, take your blood pressure, measure your hand (or foot) temperature, and monitor your heart rate. Record this information on your data sheet, and, as with earlier exercises, tally your average scores once a week.

SYSTEMATIC MUSCULAR RELAXATION (SMR) INVENTORY

Take a few moments to learn from your experience by reflecting on and answering the following questions:

Note your before-relaxation-session
    hand (foot) temperature _____
Note your after-relaxation-session
    hand (foot) temperature _____

1. By the end of SMR, had your sense of relaxation deepened?
2. Overall, how would you rate your state of relaxation on a -10 to $+10$ point scale? How does that compare to the rating you gave yourself before the relaxation exercise began?
3. Which parts of your body were easiest to relax?
4. Which parts of your body, if any, were most difficult to relax?
5. How did SMR affect your (a) blood pressure, (b) pulse and (c) hand (foot) temperature?
6. Did you notice that your hand or foot temperature increased when you relaxed specific muscular areas?
7. Did anything interfere with your practice session? If so, what could you do, if anything, to prevent this interference in the future?

To integrate SMR into your overall relaxation practice, the following sequence is recommended:

1. Begin your sessions with a reclining or standing stretch.
2. Settle into the position you have already determined is most comfortable for relaxing.
3. Once you are comfortable, deepen and extend your breathing with three minutes of the Three-Part Complete Breathing technique.
4. Move through the Systematic Muscular Relaxation sequence.
5. Focus on the autogenic phrases you have found most effective in

increasing your body peripheral warmth and subjective relaxation.

COMMON PROBLEMS DURING RELAXATION PRACTICE

Initially, you may find that some of your muscles relax only partially. Keep in mind that you will be able to relax your muscles more effectively with practice. Forcing your muscles to relax is not an effective strategy; as with warming your hands, this will paradoxically have the opposite effect, causing even more tension. Dr. David Bresler, former director of the UCLA Pain Control Unit, has compared forcing yourself to relax to forcing yourself to fall asleep or to remember a name; you just can't do it.

If you have difficulty bringing your awareness to or relaxing particular parts of your body, you may find it helpful to focus on these areas as you inhale, then feel and imagine the tension flowing out as you exhale. Use words that encourage relaxation such as "relax" and "let go." Your muscles may relax more easily if you first tighten them, then allow them to relax. Also, try practicing SMR after a hot shower, bath, or massage. Gentle sustained stretches done with awareness—such as those practiced in hatha-yoga—can help release chronically tense muscles as well.

Recognize that your muscles became tight while attempting to serve you in the "line of duty." If you find that your muscles are chronically tight, you may wish to empathize with them, letting them know that they had good reason to tighten. Accept the tension and let your muscles know it is now okay to relax. Relaxation is the process of letting go. You need to allow it to take place.

At times, you may find it difficult to adhere to a twice-a-day practice schedule. The events of the day will get in the way, and your relaxation session may seem like an expendable commitment when you are pressed for time. This is exactly the time to remind yourself of nationally-syndicated columnist Sydney J. Harris' insight, "The time to relax is when you don't have time for it."

Stan, an executive whose blood pressure was uncontrolled when he entered the HART Program, learned the benefits of regular relaxation practice. At the onset of the program, he was taking multiple antihypertensive medications, and was at particular risk because he was also a heavy smoker.

During his first few weeks in the program, Stan experienced a series of personal crises—his mother was dying, his wife's mother was also very ill, he was having problems with his teenagers, and his workload had increased. These circumstances added to his stress and further increased his blood pressure. Although he came to the clinic sessions, he practiced Systematic Muscular Relaxation and the other HART techniques only erratically during the first month. Consequently, he wasn't getting results.

When stress increases, regular relaxation sessions become even more important. I encouraged Stan to stick with the program and to use a tape at home as additional support when practicing.

A short time later, Stan began setting aside time for consistent relaxation practice, and he rapidly started to see improvements. His blood pressure declined, which increased his motivation to keep practicing regularly. His blood pressure continued to fall, eventually reaching normal levels. Under his doctor's guidance, he reduced the amount of medication he was taking, and his blood pressure readings still remained within a normal range.

There is almost always something that needs to be done, someplace to go, or some problem that can occupy your time. Carving out two 15-minute periods a day for relaxation needs to be a high priority. If you find it challenging to establish a regular twice-daily practice routine, come up with strategies to support you in getting back on course. For example, schedule your sessions in advance and honor your commitment just as you would an appointment with your doctor or a valued friend. If you can't devote two full 15-minute periods to your relaxation practice on a particular day, fit it in even in an abbreviated five- or ten-minute form. Be prepared to acknowledge the creativity of the rationalizations your mind will generate as to why you can't possibly practice on a given day, and then set them aside. Your health and well-being are counting on you.

So on days when you have ample time for your relaxation practice, do it. And on days when it just seems impossible to fit it in, do it anyway.

*Relaxation is the **natural** state of your body once you have quieted your mind and swept the tension away that can build up over days, months and years. Much of this tension can be held in our muscles, and releasing it can not only increase equanimity but also help normalize your blood pressure.*

In the next chapter, you will build upon what you have learned about relaxation, using your skills to help create vivid images that can become another important tool in controlling hypertension.

CHAPTER · 10

The Impact of Imagery

So great a power is there of the psyche upon the body, that whichever way the psyche imagines and dreams that it goes, thither doth it lead the body.

—Agrippa, 1510

When it comes to the autonomic nervous system, an image is worth a thousand words.

—adapted proverb

WHICH EXERTS A more powerful influence on your mind/body processes: the language of imagery or a verbal command? Let's find out. Close your eyes, and picture yourself holding a large, ripe, succulent, yellow lemon. Take a moment to create a vivid picture of it. Feel its weight in your hand.

Now, imagine placing your lemon on a cutting board, picking up a knife, and slicing the lemon into quarters.

Take a section of the imaginary lemon that seems particularly wet and juicy. Feel its moist skin, slightly rough texture, and coolness. Bring the lemon to your mouth and take a bite. Can you smell and taste the sour juice splashing into your mouth? Can you sense your taste buds startled by the sudden tartness of hundreds of droplets of juice? Did your lips pucker and tongue react to the sharp, pungent taste?

For the next few months, continue to focus on tasting the lemon. Squeeze a bit more juice into your mouth. Do you sense the amount of saliva in your mouth increasing?

Now, with the same goal, switch strategies. This time, rely solely on a verbal command without picturing anything in your mind. Say to yourself: "Produce saliva!" How much saliva did you generate? Maybe you were able to create a little, but perhaps barely enough to moisten your mouth. Many people can't produce any.

Were you able to generate more saliva using the pictures, taste, and tactile sensations of your full sensory imagination, or with the verbal command alone? For most of us, vivid feelings, sensations, sounds, sights, smells, and tastes evoke a greater physiological response. You may have just experienced first-hand how clear, powerful pictures and feelings constructed in your own mind can produce a desired effect on your physiology. Images are the language of the inner self.

Later in this chapter, you will see how this technique can increase the warmth of your body periphery and lower your blood pressure. And that's really not surprising. The Autonomic Nervous System (ANS) responds to imagery. Mental images are what you just used to communicate with the unconscious mechanisms that control salivation. Perhaps even more important, critical life functions ranging from your heart rate and breathing to immune function and blood pressure respond to visualization as well.

In this chapter, after further exploring the impact of imagery, we will focus on opening up your own innate imaging capacity and putting it to work to deepen your relaxation and increase your hand and foot warmth—core techniques for tuning down your sympathetic nervous system activity, expanding constricted blood vessels, and lowering blood pressure.

LETTING YOUR IMAGINATION WORK FOR YOU

Whether you realize it or not, we all think in images. Studies indicate that much of our thinking is image based, and we encode a considerable amount of information in a multisensory memory. Harvard University researchers have found that literally everyone can create some form of mental picture. You may never have experimented with the power of the images formed in your mind, since imagination is generally undervalued in our culture. Many of us tend to repress our creative and imaginative attributes in favor of our verbal and rational sides, which are more highly esteemed and rewarded.

So don't be surprised if you aren't yet aware that imaging is part of your natural thinking process, particularly since the images are often quite fleeting. With some coaching, however, everyone I work with discovers that they do indeed form images—and they learn to develop this resource as a tool for warming their body periphery, reducing their sympathetic nervous system activity, deepening their relaxation, and normalizing their blood pressure.

JUST HOW POWERFUL ARE IMAGES?

Hypertension isn't the only area in which pictures in your mind's eye can promote healing. When orthopedic surgeon Robert Swearingen treats ski-accident victims near the slopes of Colorado, he helps them relax and encourages them to imagine the healing taking place. He explains how broken bones heal and shows patients how to visualize this process occurring. When these individuals regularly practice this imagery technique, they are able to dramatically reduce their pain and the healing time they require. Dr. Swearingen has reported that casts can be removed about 30 percent earlier in patients who incorporate relaxation and visualization into their daily routine.

Norman Cousins, while an adjunct professor at the UCLA School of Medicine, helped patients recognize that they are capable of increasing blood flow to their hands as a way of freeing them from feelings of helplessness that often accompany severe illness. In *Head First: The Biology of Hope*, Cousins described patients who—through imagery and relaxation techniques—learned to raise the surface temperature of their skin at least 10 degrees. When that happens, wrote Cousins, "their entire relationship to their bodies is apt to undergo a profound change." Cousins told patients, "Medical researchers have demonstrated that we have a measure of control even over our autonomic functions. Our control is much greater than we realize. Now, move your blood into your hands. You can do it. Just visualize your heart pumping your blood up to your shoulders; now cross the shoulders; now down your arms, past the elbow, down the forearm, past the wrist, and into your hands."

When patients opened their eyes and checked their hand temperature, they usually found that it had increased significantly. After learning that they could move the blood to alter their skin temperature, these patients sometimes asked Cousins, "Did I really do it myself?" Cousins typically responded, "Yes. If you can do this, what else can you do?"

UCLA's program in psychoneuroimmunology has funded the development of a lecture series for its medical students on how to use guided imagery to improve patient care by helping individuals activate their own healing mechanisms. The program also created a film about using relaxation and visual imagery to facilitate positive mental states and attitudes and speed recovery from illness. Years earlier, the UCLA Pain Control Unit, under the direction of Dr. David Bresler, pioneered the use of relaxation and visualization in the treatment of chronic pain.

Dr. Dean Ornish, an innovative clinician and researcher who began investigating visualization at Harvard Medical School, now routinely teaches guided imagery as one means of actually reversing coronary heart disease. Using visualization in conjunction with other approaches, including proper nutrition, meditation, stress management, and exercise, patients have been able to produce significant improvements in the functioning of their heart.

In developing his program, Dr. Ornish recognized that coronary heart disease is caused by a diminished flow of blood to the heart. Thus, he postulated, the same nervous-system mechanisms that allow people to control blood flow to the hands might also influence the constriction and dilation of the arteries supplying blood to the heart.

Dr. Ornish's patients visualize removing blockages within their coronary arteries, using images such as a "bottle brush swooshing through [the] coronary arteries" or "a Roto-Rooter reaming out the blockages," as Ornish writes in *Stress, Diet, and Your Heart*. Patients also picture the healthy arteries and heart they want to create: the heart beating strongly and regularly, pumping blood efficiently and effortlessly through relaxed, dilated coronary arteries. They may visualize new arteries branching out and growing into areas of the body that required an increased blood flow. Dr. Ornish advises, "If you begin your day this way, your subconscious mind will tend to carry these healthy images throughout your day." He also encourages his patients to complete each session by seeing themselves as healthy individuals.

The pioneering work of Carl and Stephanie Simonton uses imagery as an adjunct to conventional cancer therapy. They encourage patients to relax twice daily and imagine their disease-fighting white blood cells in symbolic form—as white knights on horseback, attacking and annihilating their cancer cells. The result: A greater percentage of patients who use this visualization technique significantly increase their chances for remission and a lengthened life span. According to the Simontons, as well as researchers at the University of Texas Health Science Center, the patients who fare best are those who picture their white blood cells as Vikings or other powerful figures battling for a good cause. By contrast, patients who visualize their immune cells as soft clouds or snowflakes tend to have poor outcomes. Those who see their own healing forces as stronger than the cancer cells have a much better prognosis than those who do not.

Actively imaging a desired outcome has proven useful in other fields. In sports, many athletes have learned how to use their mind and imagination to improve their performance. For instance, when training for an important game or event, tennis players or gymnasts regularly relax and visualize in great detail every move they are going to make while hitting a backhand or performing intricate choreography on a high bar.

In essence, these athletes are programming preferred psychophysiological responses into their nervous system, thus improving the likelihood that they will excel. Their neuromuscular network is "going through the motions," although the individuals themselves may be resting comfortably at the time. The mind is learning to make the right connections with the muscles, although there appears to be no real activity going on. Karl Pribram, a Stanford researcher, has described this visualization technique as creating "mental holograms"—three-dimensional images that channel nerve impulses to the appropriate muscles.

One study found that when basketball players visualized themselves accurately shooting one basket after another, they experienced improvements in their performance equal to players who actually practiced with a real ball and basket. In a separate landmark study, top Soviet athletes were divided into four groups whose training programs varied in the following way:

Group I devoted 100 percent of its training time to physical activity.

Group II spent 75 percent of its time in physical training, and 25 percent in mental training such as imagery.

Group III divided its time 50-50 between physical and mental activities.

Group IV devoted just 25 percent of its time to physical training, spending the other 75 percent on mental training.

Researchers then compared the performance of these four groups. Group IV—the athletes who had spent the most time practicing imagery techniques—demonstrated the greatest improvement. Group III was next, followed by Groups II and I.

Visualization has clearly proven its usefulness. Mental training is a central part of the sports system not only in the USSR, but for many athletes in the United States and around the world.

IMAGERY: THE HIGHER ORDER LANGUAGE OF OUR RIGHT BRAIN

Our brain and nervous system are exquisitely complex. There are about 10 billion nerve cells within our nervous system, and each one of them has approximately 5,000 interconnections. Thus, there are almost an unlimited number of ways in which information and images can be transmitted through this network.

Although the brain has two hemispheres—left and right—imagery is the language of the right brain. This right hemisphere is intuitive, creative, emotional, and associative. We use it in activities like envisioning new ideas and strategies, playing music, and drawing. Our right brain communicates primarily through pictures and is our best means of reaching and influencing the ANS, which controls blood pressure and other physiological functions fundamental to sustaining life.

By contrast, the left hemisphere of the brain specializes in logical, rational, linear, and analytical thinking processes. Its primary communication system is verbal. We rely on the left brain to do arithmetic calculations or to carry on a conversation.

Our body's most basic functions operate without the need for constant attention: the heart pumps 2,000 gallons of blood during each 24-hour period, and respiration functions continuously, day and night. These processes occur without conscious monitoring. If, however, vigilant overseeing **were** necessary, verbal orders like, "Blood pressure, go down" wouldn't be nearly as helpful as using your right brain's capacity to generate multisensory images to influence autonomic processes. We are learning that through pictures (which are the symbolic, "higher order" language of the right brain) you *can* influence parts of your body once thought to be outside your control. Whether it is lowering blood pressure, reversing heart disease, shrinking cancerous tumors, alleviating the symptoms of illness, or healing injuries, the imagination can play a role. When it comes to the autonomic system, an image **is** "worth a thousand words."

USING IMAGING TO WARM HANDS AND LOWER BLOOD PRESSURE

As with the exercises in previous chapters, the imaging technique you will learn here is designed to relax and warm your body periphery, tune down the activity of your sympathetic nervous system, and decrease your blood pressure. Using imagery, you can calm your body and increase blood flow to the extremities—often just by imagining "hot" experiences like relaxing on the beach or warming your hands before a toasty fire.

In this process, your goal is to raise your hand temperature to 95.5 degrees; then, after you've developed some proficiency in handwarming, to focus on raising your foot temperature into the low 90s (93–95 degrees). Just as techniques like autogenic phrases, Three-Part Complete Breathing, and muscular relaxation facilitate this warming process, so can using your imagination. The goal is to be able to feel your extremities become hot within seconds, raise your hand and foot temperature to the desired levels within a minute or two, and maintain this warmth for ten minutes during your relaxation practice. This type of warming and deep relaxing breaks the stress cycle, restores your homeostasis, and lowers your blood pressure.

Some of my patients have found that vividly imagining a tranquil, natural environment that they find particularly relaxing works best for them. Others prefer the more direct, physiological approach of actually picturing the warming taking place inside their bodies. Many have discovered that combining these two approaches works most effectively. You will know what images work best for you by watching your temperature device.

Here are examples of some experiences with imagery:

Bob is a mechanical engineer. He actually thinks of his heart as a pump. He creates an image of this mechanical device channeling bright red, oxygenated, warm blood through long tubes into his limbs. As his mental picture becomes stronger, Bob feels increasing warmth flowing down his arms into his hands and fingers and down his thighs and legs into his feet and toes. As his hands and feet warm, he experiences tingling sensations in his extremities. At the same time, his hand and foot temperatures rise.

Steven visualizes sitting by a hot, burning fire, keeping his feet and hands close enough to the leaping flames so that they become toasty warm. "Sometimes I would be out at the beach next to a bonfire," he says. "Other times, the fire would be on a stove. It depends on where I choose to take my fantasy. But heat is always a part of it."

Edward is drawn to the ocean—a sight he finds particularly relaxing. He visualizes himself swimming freely underwater. "I feel myself much like a porpoise breaking through the water, completely relaxed, completely at ease." Once Edward develops this pleasant image, he shifts to one that deals specifically with warming his hands: walking up to a hot campfire on the beach, reaching his hands out so he can feel its heat, and experiencing his fingers and toes becoming warmer and warmer.

To unwind and focus, Cynthia visualizes herself walking along a path on the bank of a river, enjoying the feelings of being in motion, the beauty of the water, and the clusters of green, leafy trees. She then imagines herself jogging to an orchard and resting under sweet scented, blossoming cherry trees. As she relaxes, she enjoys the play of warm light filtering through the blossom-laden branches—and she senses her hands and feet warming.

DEVELOPING A MULTISENSORY IMAGE

Here is an example of how to develop an image for relaxation and warming your hands or feet. Visualize a beach scene. Begin by picturing yourself walking along soft, sun-drenched sands stretching along an expanse of sparkling, aquamarine water, watching and listening to the ebb and flow of waves lapping the shore. As you walk, deeply filling your lungs with the clean, fresh air, you hear a bird call and look up to see a flock of gulls rising into the sky, skimming over the water, then disappearing into the horizon. You notice how particularly warm and radiant the golden sun is, how good it feels to be here. You see palm trees in the distance.

Ready to relax, you walk up the beach to a cluster of tall green palms and make yourself comfortable on a chair beneath them. Lulled by the sound of the water, you close your eyes and notice your breath deepening and synchronizing to the slow, rhythmic rising and ebbing of the waves flowing onto the shore and retreating into the vast ocean. You might even imagine that your breath is like a wave of the ocean: as you inhale, the wave is flowing in and through you from your toes to your head, and as you exhale, it flows out again, revitalizing and relaxing you, more and more deeply.

It feels so good to recline under the warm sun as it filters down between the palm fronds swaying gently in the tropical breeze. As you relax even more deeply, you grow aware of your hands and feet becoming even warmer as rays of sunshine stream down upon them.

What you've just experienced is multisensory imagery, where you don't just **see** the scene in your mind's eye, you also **feel** your relaxation deepen, your hand and foot temperatures rise, and you *experience* the sounds, smells, and tastes around you. Some people find that instead of experiencing the scene directly, they seem to be watching themselves from an observer's position. This is not as effective. If it happens with you, just imagine stepping back into your body to make your experience more immediate and tangible.

As you practice, you may find that one of your senses in your experience is more vivid than the others. Take whichever one is most tangible for you and build upon it in a process called "overlapping," which means adding your other senses one at a time. Don't just **look** at your surroundings and the source of your warmth, but **feel** the warming take place, **listen** to the sounds and experience the **smells** that could be around you. Be there as fully as you can.

Applying this to the image we just developed, we can add to the richness of the experience by not only seeing the sights on a beach, but also by getting in touch with the feeling of the soft warm sand, the sound of the waves flowing onto the shore and then retreating back into the ocean, the call of the seagulls soaring through the sky, the fresh taste and smell of the salt air, and our hands and feet growing hot as we bask in the warm sun. Start with the aspect of the scene or your experience that you can create most clearly, then built upon it, bringing in what you perceive through your other senses. You will soon have a more complete representation of what it is like to actually be relaxing and practicing your hand/foot warming at the beach or wherever you choose to be.

During this exercise, as you focus on the warming process, you might also bring in a more anatomical image of the warming that is occurring, allowing yourself to feel and see your blood vessels relaxing and expanding as your blood flows smoothly and easily through your circulatory system down your arms into your hands, and down your legs into your toes. As your blood moves to your hands and feet, they may begin to feel heavier and warmer and start to tingle or pulse, further deepening your relaxation and increasing your hand and foot temperature.

GETTING STARTED

To begin the imaging process, find a quiet place where you won't be disturbed. As with the exercises in earlier chapters, measure your blood pressure, pulse rate, and finger (or toe) temperature. By using a small thermometer (or other temperature monitoring device) during these sessions, you will be able to monitor the changes in your peripheral body temperature, which will help you discover those images most effective in increasing your hand or foot warmth.

Again, here is what you can expect: By raising your hand temperature to 95.5 degrees and your foot temperature to 93 degrees, you will shift your sympathetic nervous system from a state of overactivation to one of relaxation. As that happens, your blood vessel walls will dilate, permitting greater circulation, which in turn results in increased hand and foot warmth.

During the imaging process, to get feedback on how well you are warming your extremities, you might want to glance occasionally at the thermometer to see if your hand or foot temperature is increasing. Be sure to do this in a relaxed manner; that is, through half-closed eyes and with an objective frame of mind. Remember that intending and allowing warming to occur—and seeing and feeling the warming take place—is much more effective than actively striving to warm your hands and feet or demanding that they warm, which will most likely result in cooling them.

While some individuals I work with develop imaging best through relaxing and creating their own visualization, others benefit from a more structured approach, perhaps even prescripting their visualization. This can be particularly helpful in the beginning.

What follows is a set of instructions to lead you through the process of creating your own multisensory image for relaxing and warming your body periphery. You might decide to have a friend or family member read these instructions to you as you go through them, or you can record them onto a cassette tape and then play them back as you practice. While the following transcript can be helpful when you start, you will no longer need it once you have successfully launched your own imaging process.

As in your regular practice sessions, be sure to measure and write down your preimaging (or prerelaxation) hand and foot temperature, blood pressure, and pulse. To integrate imagery into your overall relaxation practice, the following sequence is best:

1. Begin your sessions with a reclining or standing stretch.
2. Settle into the position you have determined is most comfortable for relaxing.
3. Once you are comfortable, deepen and extend your breathing with three minutes of the Three-Part Complete Breathing technique.
4. Proceed through the Systematic Muscular Relaxation sequence.
5. As you develop your imagery, you may wish to intersperse it with the particular autogenic phrases that were most effective for quieting your body, mind, and emotions, and warming your hands and feet. Select these phrases in advance and write them down to incorporate them into your session.

CREATING A MULTISENSORY IMAGE FOR RELAXATION AND WARMING YOUR HANDS AND FEET

1. Stretch, settle into a comfortable position, and focus your attention on your breathing.
2. For the next few minutes, deepen and extend your breath with the Three-Part Complete Breathing technique.
3. Relax your muscles from feet to head with Systematic Muscular Relaxation.
4. Note your hand or foot temperature. As you relax, allow your awareness to move inward and your mind, body and emotions to become calm . . . quiet . . . at ease . . . and relaxed. With each long and deep breath, you will move more fully into a right-brain mode in which it's easier to generate imagery.

   Most of us know, or, with brief reverie, will discover the place where we feel most relaxed and at ease—the place we might want to go in our mind's eye when we feel most in need of restoration or recreation. Imagine being in your favorite tranquil environment. It can be an actual place or one that you create. What counts is that it is the place **you** want to be. Take a few minutes to explore the place you have chosen. Start with whatever image looks, feels, or sounds right to you, then develop your experience from there. What is it like? What can you see, feel, and hear in this special place?

5. Note your peripheral body temperature again. For some people, imaging occurs instantly, incorporating every major sense. For most of us, however, visualization takes practice and development. Accept the sensory impression that comes most easily for you—whether it is what you see, feel, or hear. Use this impression to overlap or bridge into your other senses. For the next few minutes, discover and develop the details of what you can see, feel, and hear around you that will enhance your sense of tranquility, calm, warming, and well-being.

   Focusing on what you create will make your visualization more tangible, further deepening your relaxation and increasing your hand and foot warmth.

   What feelings does being in this special place evoke? Perhaps a greater sense of calm or serenity? Let whatever positive feelings you can experience by being here increase.

6. Note your temperature. What do you see around you? Discover details in your surroundings that are pleasing to you. As you do so, imagine them becoming brighter and more vivid . . . .

   What bodily or tactile sensations are you now aware of that can add to your comfort? How does your experience evoke a greater sense of relaxation and warmth? As you become aware of these or other feelings of comfort you may be experiencing, allow them to become more tangible and feel your relaxation deepen.

7. Glance at your temperature again. What naturally-occurring sounds are contributing to your relaxation and enjoyment? As you tune in to these sounds around you, note how they become more audible . . . . Can you detect any scent or taste that is part of your environment?

8. Note your temperature. What is the source of warmth in your image? Allow it to grow brighter and warmer. Do you sense your hands or feet becoming warmer? What does this increasing warmth feel or look like? As your relaxation deepens, perhaps you can imagine seeing and feeling the warm flow of circulation moving from your heart, across your shoulders, down your arms and into your hands. Or perhaps you can see and feel warmth flowing from your heart, down into your torso and legs, and into your feet. As your hands and feet get warmer, feel your vasculature relaxing and expanding, thereby increasing the ease with which your blood circulates to your body periphery and causing your hands and feet to get even warmer. Perhaps you feel a pulsing and tingling. Imagine your blood flowing efficiently and freely through relaxed, dilated

arteries, and your hands and feet continuing to warm with the increased flow of warm blood.

9. For the next few minutes, continue with your imagery. As you relax more deeply, feel your hands and feet becoming even warmer. Imagine yourself and your cardiovascular system as perfectly healthy. Note your temperature.

10. Before concluding your imaging session, take a few moments to be aware of the place you have created in your mind ... what you see ... how you feel ... your bodily sensations as you relax more deeply ... your hands and feet getting warmer.

This special inner place you have created is now part of your own private "channel" for relaxation. You will be able to switch it on and tune it in instantly by simply closing your eyes and being there. Once you are able to do so, you can immediately begin focusing on warming your hands and feet. Each time you relax in this special place, you'll feel better and your skills will get stronger.

As you bring your session to completion, take a deep breath. Feeling relaxed, refreshed, and revitalized, enjoy a lengthy stretch. When you are ready, open your eyes.

When you have finished your visualization session, check and record your hand or foot temperature, take your blood pressure, and measure your pulse rate. Compare these readings with the ones you obtained at the beginning of the session.

Note your thoughts and feelings about the visualization process. If it was anything less than enjoyable and relaxing, think about how to change it to your satisfaction. Was your experience vivid and tangible? Are there aspects of it you could develop further? Did your experience include feelings of warmth, sounds, sights, smells, tastes, and touch? Did you find certain parts of it particularly enjoyable or surprising?

Take a few minutes to answer the questions in the Imaging Inventory, which follows. This guide should provide you with additional insights to help you develop your skills.

IMAGING INVENTORY FOR WARMING YOUR HANDS AND FEET

1. What changes in your hand (or foot) temperature did you observe during your session? Did the temperature increase, decrease, or stay the same?
2. What in your experience may have influenced these changes? Respond as specifically as you can.
   a. Describe what you saw that may have increased (decreased) your hand or foot temperature.
   b. Describe any feelings or thoughts that may have increased (or decreased) your hand or foot temperature.
   c. Describe any bodily, tactile, or internal sensations that may have increased (or decreased) your hand or foot temperature.
   d. Did you experience any sense of warmth, flowing, pulsing, or tingling? Did any other feelings accompany your increase in hand or foot temperature (such as increased relaxation or tranquility)?
3. Describe the source(s) of warmth in your imaging experience.
4. What, if anything, could you do to increase your effectiveness in using imaging for warming your hands or feet?
5. What, if anything, may have interfered with your session? What could you do in the future to prevent such disturbances?

Periodically review the following seven pointers for effective imaging.

SEVEN POINTERS FOR EFFECTIVE IMAGING

The objective of imaging is to assist you in relaxing and warming your hands to 95.5 degrees. Once you have developed this ability, switch to warming your feet to 93 degrees. With practice, and by following these pointers, you will be able to warm your hands and feet almost instantaneously and learn to maintain warmer hand and foot temperatures during your relaxation sessions.

1. Intermittently check your thermometer (or other temperature monitoring device) during your session to learn what images may be affecting your hand (or foot) temperature. Use this information to develop your skills.
2. Remember, intending to warm your body periphery, seeing/ feeling the warming occurring, and allowing your hand (foot) temperature to increase will facilitate warming. Worrying about,

insisting on, or verbally commanding the warming to occur will only have the opposite effect.

3. Incorporate all five senses into your imaging process as much as possible. Start with your most dominant sense (the one you generate most easily), then overlap or bridge into the other senses. Become aware of each sense in turn, incorporating them one at a time, into your image. Paying attention to the details of your experience will help you sustain and deepen your focus and increase the effectiveness of the imaging process.

4. Include a source of warmth in your imaging process. Develop a visual image to represent your hand (or foot) temperature increasing.

5. Be aware of your own subjective sensations (namely, warmth, flowing, tingling, pulsing), and allow them to intensify. As these sensations become stronger, your temperature will rise. You will be able to use these same sensations to increase hand and foot warmth specifically.

6. Some people choose to write their images down, then transfer them to a tape they can use as a guide in future practice sessions. If you decide to do this, use graphic, sensory-based language, and include even the small details. Use short sentences; the more vivid and tangible, the better. Alternate using your tape and imaging on your own until you have successfully mastered the imaging process.

7. Practice and develop your imaging and warming techniques as part of your twice-a-day relaxation periods. Remember that learning any new skill takes practice. While some individuals see substantial increases in temperature during their first session, others take a few sessions before they find the images that work best for them. Learn from your experience. Warming up to relax will soon become second-nature.

Strategies for Applying Stress Management Skills in Daily Life: Constant Instant Practice

In being able to handle stress, I am 150 degrees different from where I started. Initially, anything would have me going into orbit. But now when I'm in stressful situations, I'm able to identify stress and control it.

> —MARK
> Oil company executive
> Hart participant

Take a rest, a field that has rested gives a bountiful crop.

> —OVID
> Roman poet
> 1st century A.D.

SINCE STRESS CAN be a frequent and even continuous part of our lives, our health and well-being rest on whether we can appraise and manage it constructively on a daily basis. Up to now, you have been learning how to use the self-regulatory skills of the HART Program to control your hypertension. In this second phase of the program you will be continuing with your extended, twice-daily relaxation practice, while also learning to instantly use your relaxation skills, in an abbreviated form at frequent intervals during your day. Developing instant access to these techniques will enable you to maintain or more rapidly reestablish your inner balance when your response to a stressor threatens to disrupt the equilibrium or homeostasis you have been working so hard to achieve. This process you will learn, called Constant Instant Practice (CIP), will help you successfully regulate your blood pressure for life by altering your established patterns for dealing with day-to-day stressors, teaching you new, more constructive ways of managing stress.

THE IMPORTANCE OF STRESS MANAGEMENT

Thus far, you have only been measuring your blood pressure before and after your relaxation sessions. Now you will see that it is also important to be aware of how your blood pressure behaves in response to the stressful situations of everyday life.

If you're like many people, you may respond to stressful situations by getting angry or frustrated, and allowing those feelings to build up until they translate into significant rises in blood pressure. Even your reaction to minor irritants—such as waiting at traffic lights, losing your keys, or dealing with slow service at a restaurant—can activate your sympathetic nervous system, which in turn can cause blood pressure to spike. Some studies, using portable blood pressure monitoring devices along with personal stress logs, show that sudden blood pressure increases can happen 50 to 100 times a day. These sudden increases can, over time, contribute to blood pressure rising even higher, and cause additional wear upon the heart and vessel walls.

Research by Dr. Chandra Patel, a pioneer in the development of the biobehavioral treatment for essential hypertension, underscores the importance of stress management. She put 32 hypertensive patients through two stress tests that caused their blood pressure to rise significantly, then she continued monitoring their blood pressure until their readings returned to their initial plateaus.

Dr. Patel then divided these patients into two groups, teaching only one of them the techniques that would help them relax and control their stress response. Six weeks later, she repeated the stress tests and measured blood pressure. Dr. Patel found that the people who had learned stress management and relaxation skills experienced lower jumps in blood pressure when subjected to stress, and that their blood pressure returned to normal much more quickly.

If your baseline blood pressure is already higher than normal, you especially need to alter the way you react to stress. While it is neither possible nor desirable to lead a life completely without stress, new and healthier ways of responding to it can be a real asset.

Kenneth Pelletier, Ph.D., a leading authority on stress, has said that one of the distinguishing characteristics of individuals who manage stress well—and even thrive on it—is that they have learned to create "regular islands of peace" in their daily life. This can occur not only through longer relaxation sessions that bring their body/mind back to a state of homeostasis or balance, but also by frequently finding brief moments of relaxation in the context of their lives, or very short periods of relaxation in the midst of everyday challenges. Constant Instant Practice (CIP) is such a process.

WHAT IS CONSTANT INSTANT PRACTICE?

Constant Instant Practice (CIP) is essentially a three-part process that rapidly reestablishes your equilibrium in just a few moments. The aim of CIP is to break the stress cycle at its source. The CIP strategy involves three skills that you are already well-acquainted with:

1. Deepening your breathing.
2. Relaxing your muscles.
3. Warming your hands.

By using these steps, you will be developing a powerful stress-management tool for maintaining or rapidly regaining a balance of body, mind and emotions. As you implement CIP, you will be in a better position to pause, access the situation or stressor at hand, and select the best option for dealing with it most effectively—whether that means "going with the flow," or engaging in active, solution-oriented behavior. Rather than reacting to stressors with old, habitual, less-than-constructive patterns that can raise your blood pressure, obscure your best judgment, and erode your well-being, CIP can help you exercise greater freedom of choice in how you will act.

CONSTANT INSTANT PRACTICE: BREAKING THE CYCLE AT ITS SOURCE

The goal of Constant Instant Practice is to instantly break the stress cycle at its source in the course of daily life. Here are the three basic steps of CIP:

1. **Deepen Your Breathing.** The instant you detect a stressor, extend and deepen your breathing. Uninterrupted breathing—and breathing smoothly, deeply and evenly—are keys to stress control. Because your posture can affect the ease with which you breathe, gently align your body as you deepen your breathing. Deepening and extending your breathing helps override a tendency many people have to hold their breath for a few seconds or more at the onset of a stressor. Holding the breath—as well as shallow, arrhythmic, or thoracic breathing—can initiate as well as perpetuate a cascade of stressful feelings and thoughts.
2. **Relax Your Muscles.** To rapidly relax your muscles, move your awareness through your body in a wave from head to foot, simultaneously scanning for and releasing any unneeded tension or tightness. This can counter your body's tendency to brace

or tighten under stress. In addition to relaxing your muscles, give extra attention to releasing tightness in any parts of your body (such as shoulders, back, and jaw) that you discover chronically tighten under stress.

3. **Warm Your Hands.** Use the methods you have found most effective for increasing your body periphery temperature to 95.5–96 degrees—whether it is a phrase; bodily sensations (pulsing, throbbing, tingling); an image of the warming occurring in your favorite environment; a combination of these skills that you have found effective; or merely intending your hands to warm and allowing it to happen. Warming your hands as part of CIP will decrease sympathetic nervous system activity and vasodilate the arteries that contract in response to stress.

WHAT ARE YOUR SIGNS OF STRESS?

The earlier you detect stress, the easier it is to diffuse. Thus, it is essential for you to be able to recognize how you respond to stress, particularly, the initial signs of the stress response, as well as the symptoms you develop under prolonged stress. In the early part of this century, Harvard professors Robert Yerkes and John Dodson devised the so-called "Yerkes-Dodson Law," in which they emphasized that some stress is essential for good performance. A certain level of stress can create motivation and keep the creative juices flowing, providing the challenges that are a natural part of enjoying and excelling in life. When stress occurs at a manageable level, people often feel more energized and they describe making decisions more efficiently. However, when there is too much stress in life, many individuals feel overburdened and their productivity and health can suffer.

Edward, a HART participant, noticed that during his morning train commute, his internal "motor" would often seem to be running as fast as the train itself. "Until the HART Program, I never realized it," he said. "But I gradually began to recognize how anxious I felt about getting the day started, worrying about it and becoming very nervous while I rode to work."

As Edward paid attention to how he was responding, he started using his CIP stress management skills (deepening his breathing, relaxing his muscles, and warming his hands). He used his own internal signals of stress as a catalyst to practice CIP. "My body learned how to take back control very quickly," said Edward. "It was like riding a bicycle; my body seemed to know just what to do. I'd catch myself, do some deep breathing, calm down, and stop the whole stress cycle."

Barbara, another HART patient, recounted a phone conversation with a client who was acting quite unreasonably.

He was yelling, and even though I would have liked to yell back, it just wouldn't have been appropriate from a business point of view. I defended myself, but not too vigorously. I sat back and talked to him as calmly as possible. But as the minutes passed, I could tell I was getting more stressed. My hands were shaking. I could feel my heart pounding. My entire phys-iology was racing.

As Barbara sensed the changes within her own body, she used it as an opportunity to practice stress management. "While the conversation continued, I began taking deep breaths . . . relaxing my muscles . . . and warming my hands," she said. "After the phone conversation, I went through the steps of CIP again. The deep breathing in particular seemed to help a lot. I felt so much better."

Barbara was able to detect the signs of stress in her own body and take constructive action, implementing CIP to curtail a longer-term stress reaction. She was also wise enough to take steps to more fully regain her equilibrium after the tense interaction. As her skills at iden-tifying and diffusing stressful situations continued to improve, she was able to detect a stressful event even earlier and use her skills to better maintain her balance.

George, a participant in his mid-seventies, recognizes that he is about to have a stress response when he feels an increase in muscle tension in the pit of his stomach and in his shoulders. "I feel myself sort of getting churned up or excited and something kicks in—the relaxation response or something that says 'calm down, relax.' It enables me to have better control of my emotions, my feelings."

George says that in the past, he would become very angry in difficult situations and therefore he couldn't think.

I would flare up, and could literally feel my heart start pumping and my face flush. Yet with CIP and the relaxation technique, I never get that angry and I'm able to calm down. I really had problems doing that in the past because I tended to be obsessive. Now I handle those moments better. I can stay on par with the people I'm talking to without losing my train of thought or letting my anger mess up my thinking.

COMMON SIGNS OF STRESS

To break the stress cycle, it is important to be able to recognize the signs of stress. Here is a list of the most common indicators of stress. Place a check by the symptoms you sometimes feel. All of them may be stress-related. Keep in mind, however, that some of these symptoms can have other medical causes; thus, it is important to discuss your symptoms with your physician to determine whether they require treatment other than stress management.

Physical symptoms

_____ Muscular tightness   _____ Sweaty palms

_____ Increased heart rate   _____ Vomiting, nausea

_____ Cold hands and feet   _____ Over- or undereating

_____ Chest tightness   _____ Headaches

_____ Trembling, twitching   _____ Sleep disturbances

_____ Poor posture   _____ Loss of sex drive

_____ Fatigue   _____ Diarrhea or constipation

_____ Itching

_____ Difficulty breathing

Mental symptoms

_____ Poor memory   _____ Poor concentration

_____ Mistakes in grammar   _____ Absence of interests

_____ Decreased productivity   _____ Poor awareness of external stimuli

_____ Forgetfulness

Emotional symptoms

_____ Depression   _____ Impatience

_____ Outbursts of anger   _____ Irritability

_____ Anxiety   _____ Reclusiveness

_____ Lack of initiative   _____ Crying spells

_____ Self-deprecation

MAKING CIP A PART OF YOUR LIFE

As stated earlier, the objective of this part of the program is to transfer your skills to daily life by taking a few moments each hour to relax and implement CIP, as well as to use it even more frequently in stressful situations. However, there is also a longer-term goal of CIP—namely, to integrate it into your regular, day-to-day behavior. Changing your response to stress is a key to attaining desirable blood pressure results that persist over time. Integrating CIP into your life may sound simple, but it requires a good game plan and consistent follow-through.

FIVE STRATEGIES FOR APPLYING CIP IN DAILY LIFE _____

1. Do CIP for a few moments each hour, and more often in stressful situations.
2. Link CIP to specific, regularly-occurring behavioral and environmental cues.
3. Keep a CIP Daily Stress Management Log and use temperature feedback to monitor your CIP achievements.
4. Develop a list of regularly-occurring stressors in your life, and select two or three each week with which to use as opportunities to do CIP.
5. Use constructive self-talk and mental rehearsal to assist you in incorporating CIP and managing stress more effectively.

Let's look at each of the five strategies in more depth:

STRATEGY I: DO CIP HOURLY AND MORE OFTEN IN STRESSFUL SITUATIONS

This strategy is fairly straightforward: Spend a few moments each hour deepening your breathing, relaxing your muscles, and warming your hands. Pause a few moments right now to practice CIP and relax. Start off by doing CIP at times when you are not very busy or under too much stress. This will make it easier to transfer your skills to more stressful situations. Practice CIP more frequently in stressful situations.

STRATEGY II: LINK CIP TO REPEATED BEHAVIORAL AND ENVIRONMENTAL CUES

To help you remember to use CIP frequently, you may find it helpful to select two or three actions you perform regularly or things that occur in your environment as cues to use CIP. Here are some examples that HART patients have found productive:

1. **Stopping at red lights.** If red lights have been a source of irritation or impatience for you, they can serve not only as an excellent cue, but also as a minor stressor that gives you an opportunity for CIP. Several individuals who use this cue have actually started slowing down rather than racing through yellow lights so they will have an opportunity to take their foot off the accelerator and relax during the red light.

2. **Looking at your watch.** Many people respond to time pressure by becoming tense and by nervously looking at their watch or a clock. This glance at the time can become a useful reminder to deepen your breathing, relax your muscles, and warm your hands.

3. **Brushing your teeth.** Most people brush their teeth at least twice a day, so this is an excellent CIP cue. Before or after brushing your teeth, pause, relax, and take a respite from your activities for CIP.

   If you happen to be looking in the mirror as you begin your CIP, take the opportunity to smile at yourself and think of something pleasant.

4. **Eating.** Mealtimes—breakfast, lunch, dinner, and, if you wish, snacks—are excellent, periodic reminders to do CIP. Taking a few moments for CIP before you eat has the added benefit of slowing you down and reestablishing an inner balance and quiet. This will also allow you to appreciate and be more conscious of the food you are eating and, if you are sharing a meal, the company you are with.

5. **Using the telephone.** Rather than picking up an incoming call on the first ring, use the first two rings to deepen your breathing, relax your muscles, and warm your hands—then answer the phone on the third ring. If you wish, continue to relax during your phone call.

   In the same way, take a few moments for CIP **before** making phone calls, too.

6. **Putting a key into a door lock.** Some people feel strained when they depart from or return to their home or work environment. Pausing for CIP before locking or unlocking the door can serve an important purpose: reminding you to take a few moments to provide a brief island of peace to rebalance and replenish yourself so that you can meet your challenges and responsibilities with more equanimity.

Now that you are more familiar with cues, take a few minutes to think of some CIP cues that are relevant to your own lifestyle. If they work out, use them for the duration of this program; if not, select others you may find more effective. Practice using your cues at the first possible opportunity and as frequently as possible.

One other suggestion: Place a small, colored, adhesive-backed dot on your steering wheel, watch, phone, or other everyday object. This will remind you to do CIP each time you see it.

STRATEGY III. KEEP A CIP STRESS MANAGEMENT LOG AND USE TEMPERATURE FEEDBACK

Keeping a CIP Stress Management log will help you identify the situations in which you become stressed, motivate you to apply CIP in these situations, and help you monitor how well you're doing in diffusing the stress response.

You can do CIP—and use the CIP log—with or without a temperature feedback device (such as a temperature feedback ring). If you do not use a thermal feedback device, make sure you use the subjective, tension-relaxation rating scale in the log.

Let's look at how to incorporate the log into your stress management practice. Note the number of times you use CIP each hour in the column titled *Hourly Use of CIP*. Place a check in this box each time you practice.

In the next column, *Stressor*, note any specific, stressful thoughts, feelings or situations that occur in that hour. For example: "8:00— tense, stuck in traffic jam."

If you are using a temperature feedback device, note and record your hand temperature in the *Objective Temperature Change* column before your CIP.

If you are not using such a device, or, in addition to it, record your subjective level of tension or relaxation (on a −10 to +10 rating scale) in the *Subjective Change* column. You are probably already familiar with this scale, since it is part of your Daily Blood Pressure Log: −10 represents feeling completely tense, +10 completely relaxed, −1 slightly tense, and +1 slightly relaxed.

After your CIP—once you have deepened your breath, relaxed your muscles, warmed your hands, then given your body time to respond— you can return to the chart and make a few more entries. First, check your temperature ring and record your *After CIP* hand temperature. Next, determine your subjective sense of relaxation or tension and write down the number that best represents how you feel in the appropriate column.

Finally, under the *Insights and Observations* column, jot down any information that you could use to increase the effectiveness of your CIP session—signs of stress (tension in the neck or back); images or phrases that helped you manage stress better or warm your hands more effec-

H.A.R.T. CIP STRESS MANAGEMENT LOG

CIP Strategies

1. Practice CIP hourly and more frequently in stressful situations.
2. Use cues as reminder to practice CIP.
3. Use stressful situations as opportunities to implement CIP goals.

4. Use mental rehersal to assist you in implemernting CIP goals.
5. Review your goals daily, use your skills frequently. Take a few minutes each day to observe how your performance matches your goals.
6. Acknowledge/praise yourself for using CIP skills.

DAY _____ DATE _____

TIME	HOURLY USE OF CIP	STRESSOR	TEMPERATURE		SUBJECTIVE LEVEL Tension -10 Relaxation 0 +10		INSIGHTS AND OBSERVATIONS
			Before	After	Before	After	
6:00							
7:00							
8:00							
9:00							
10:00							
11:00							
12:00							
1:00							
2:00							
3:00							
4:00							
5:00							
6:00							
7:00							
8:00							
9:00							
10:00							
11:00							
12:00							

Summary Observations:

NOTE: For an enlarged, two-page spread of this chart, see Appendix 11, pp. 254-255.

tively ("Relax, it's not worth reacting to"); or observed improvements ("Much calmer this week").

Review your CIP Stress Management Log on the days you use it, noting how often you use CIP, your progress in managing stressors in general, and the specific stressors you have chosen to use as opportunities to implement CIP. Keep your CIP log for at least three to five days each week for the duration of your stress management training. To successfully use CIP, review your goals daily, use your skills frequently, and take a few minutes to observe how your performance matches your goals. Regularly acknowledge your progress in the desired direction.

Using a Temperature Feedback Ring

A thermal feedback ring or biotic band can be a helpful addition to your CIP session. This simple device is placed around your finger and worn throughout the day to give you immediate objective feedback on the state of activation or relaxation of your sympathetic nervous system. By quickly glancing at the lighted dot on your ring or band, you'll know whether your physiology is relaxed or if you are reacting to a stressor with an increase in sympathetic nervous system activity and a dip in temperature.

Declines in temperature not due to the environment signal a stress response, whereas increases in temperature let you know when you are relaxing your sympathetic nervous system. As you recall, 95.5 to 96 degrees Fahrenheit indicates a deeply relaxed state.

HART participant George found the temperature feedback ring extremely useful. "During my workday, when I felt things were getting hectic, the ring would catch my eye and would remind me of CIP," he said. "I'd say to myself, 'Let's see if I can get my hands warm.' I'd put CIP into practice, and it was remarkable watching the colors on the ring change and knowing that my hands were warming. At the same time, I knew it was good for my blood pressure and overall health."

You can purchase a thermal feedback ring or biotic band at many medical supply stores. Make sure the ring you buy shows small gradations in temperature and spans a temperature range from at least 70 to 97 degrees Fahrenheit.

What follows are general guidelines for using the most common types of thermal feedback (liquid crystal) rings. *Be sure to read the instructions on your particular model since they may vary.*

Temperature increases as you go clockwise around the dial of the ring. As temperatures rise or fall, the ring reflects these changes by illuminating different dots. The colors of these dots—from coolest to warmest—are copper, yellow, green, blue-green, and blue. Each dot represents about a two-degree increase in hand temperature. As different dots are illuminated, you can determine changes in your hand temperature.

Wear your temperature ring or biotic band during waking hours. When you are in an optimally-relaxed state, the dot at the 12:00 position lights up in a dark blue color (95 degrees), or the dot in the center of the ring—the "bull's-eye"—lights up, indicating a hand temperature of between 95 and 97 degrees.

Your goal is to maintain warmer hand temperatures as much as possible. Whenever you notice a decrease in temperature—for example, down to 85 degrees in a stressful situation—deepen your breathing, relax your muscles, and warm your hands to ease the overactivation of your sympathetic nervous system. Use the feedback from your ring or biotic band as a catalyst for implementing CIP and monitoring the process of bringing yourself back into balance.

Your thermal ring or biotic band can be extremely useful in providing objective temperature feedback for your stress management practice. Before starting CIP, figure out your hand temperature by referring to the color of the illuminated dot and its position of the ring. Then look at the chart below. Move across the top column, finding the corresponding color on your ring—copper, yellow, green, blue-green, or blue. (If more than one dot is lit, choose the last one going clockwise.) Next, going down the left-hand column, find the hour position that was lit on your ring—from 1 to 12. Then, by moving across and down the page, locate the point where these two values intersect.

USING YOUR THERMAL RING TO FIND HAND TEMPERATURE

hour	copper	yellow	green	blue-green	blue
1	67°	68.5°	70°	71.5°	73°
2	73°	73.5°	74°	74.5°	75°
3	75°	75.5°	76°	76.5°	77°
4	77°	77.5°	78°	78.5°	79°
5	79°	79.5°	80°	80.5°	81°
6	81°	81.5°	82°	82.5°	83°
7	83°	83.5°	84°	84.5°	85°
8	85°	85.5°	86°	86.5°	87°
9	87°	87.5°	88°	88.5°	89°
10	89°	89.5°	90°	90.5°	91°
11	91°	91.5°	92°	92.5°	93°
12	93°	93.5°	94°	94.5°	95°
center Δ	95°	95.5°	96°	96.5°	97

Write this temperature down in the *Before CIP* column of your Stress Management log. Then start CIP. Allow time for your body to respond, then check your feedback ring again. With the help of the chart, see if any changes have occurred, and write down your current hand temperature in the *After CIP* column. Again, the object is to learn to warm your hands to 95 or 96 degrees within a minute or two.

STRATEGY IV: DEVELOP A LIST OF REGULARLY-OCCURRING STRESSORS TO USE AS OPPORTUNITIES TO DO CIP

Let's take a moment to look at the stressors in your life and how you respond to them. More than likely, there are certain events that routinely trigger your stress response. Your reaction to them may have become habitual over the years. With practice, however, you can learn healthier ways of responding.

The common stressors in your life are those events or situations, thoughts and feelings that "make you" tense, impatient, excited, concerned, angry, upset, depressed, anxious, frustrated, or just plain irritated. They may be related to work, relationships with family or friends, health, bills, your home, or the car. They can range from small irritants and hassles to major, demanding life changes. Stressors can also be events you enjoy or are happy about, but that require some adjustment or adaptation—such as moving, a job promotion, new relationship, or having a baby.

Even the little insults of life can take a toll. As American playwright Clifford Odets noted, "Just about anybody can face a crisis . . . . Everyday living is rough."

Most of us have no shortage of stressors. Take a few minutes right now to list the current stressors in your life; 15 to 20 stressful situations you regularly encounter. First list the more minor, "garden variety" stressors. You might be surprised at how many you can come up with. Next, make a list of the moderate stressors you encounter, followed by a few of the larger ones.

Once you have completed your list, order the items on it from the least to the most stressful. Mark the least stressful number 1—for example, stopping at a red light or getting stuck in traffic. The intermediate stressors should come next (perhaps your kids or your housemate not doing their share of the workload at home, or maybe an extra job assignment that you must complete at home at night). Finally, add your larger stressors, such as giving an important presentation at work.

In the upcoming week, focus your attention on the first two or three of these events—the most minor, least stressful ones on your list. By starting with the mildest stressors and learning to deal effectively with them, you will build your skills for tackling the more challenging problems later.

During this first week, whenever any one of the first two or three situations occurs, consciously implement CIP to short-circuit the stress response. For example, let's say that you're the type of person who fumes each time your car gets caught at a long red light. Unconsciously, your shoulders tighten, your hands clench the steering wheel, you utter expletives, and then hold your breath until the light changes. It is time to alter your reaction: Loosen your grip on the steering wheel, take a few deep breaths, allow your shoulders to drop down from around your ears, relax your muscles in a wave from head to toe—and allow your hands to warm. Feel the tension dissolve as you relax.

In the few seconds before the traffic light changes, you'll notice equilibrium replacing the stress response; CIP will help bring your body-mind into balance.

As you might expect, it can be difficult to use CIP in some situations, whether they are mildly stressful or in "the heat of battle." However, even if you are unable to diffuse the stress response at its onset, use your skills after the fact to bring yourself back into a more balanced state.

A HART patient named Todd described a stressful contract renegotiation in which he was a central player. For an intense hour, he was on the phone, trying to find a meeting of minds to resolve one difficult issue after another. "I could really feel my adrenaline pumping, and barely had time to catch my breath," he said.

Todd described how he leaned back, took some deep breaths, and allowed his body to relax. Then he took a couple minutes to walk outside and stretch. He rapidly recaptured a sense of calm so he could productively make use of the rest of his workday.

By cutting short the duration and intensity of the stress response, Todd minimized its consequences. "CIP doesn't take a lot of time," he said. "For me, even a few moments makes a big difference."

CIP can work very quickly. Even just a few seconds—the time it takes for a traffic signal to turn from red to green—can be sufficient to relax and break the stress cycle.

After your first week of CIP, move on to the next two or three stressors from your list. Again, whenever these events occur, use CIP to intercept the stress response. You may want to make use of the Guidelines for Specifying Your Weekly CIP Goals to help you select and specify your CIP goals for stressors that you find especially challenging.

GUIDELINES FOR SPECIFYING YOUR WEEKLY CIP GOALS ——

1. Briefly describe the stressful situation in which you want to use your CIP skills.
2. Describe the best way to respond to this situation. What specific skills do you want to develop or use more frequently in this situation?
3. Describe how you used to respond to this situation.
4. How will your stress management skills positively affect you or others who may be involved?
5. What will you see, hear, and feel first that will signal an opportunity to use your preferred skills?

STRATEGY V: USE CONSTRUCTIVE SELF-TALK AND MENTAL REHEARSAL TO ASSIST YOU IN INCORPORATING CIP AND MANAGING STRESS MORE EFFECTIVELY

How we perceive and appraise a situation, and what we tell ourselves about how it will affect us, are keys to whether we will respond with more balance and sense of control, or become stressed and experience an alarm response. In the first part of this strategy—constructive self-talk—the goal is to develop statements to say to yourself during times of stress that will help you manage the stress better. This internal dialogue, in tandem with your other CIP skills, will assist you in getting your body-mind back into a state of balance and equilibrium.

Many individuals have found the following phrases useful:

1. Feeling stressed is not going to help this situation.
2. Listen to me—you can *do* it.
3. I'll just get started and then I'll be all right.
4. Take things one step at a time. Everything will be fine.
5. Relax . . . be calm.
6. Problems are an opportunity to engage in solution-oriented behavior.
7. I've done this before and I can do it again.
8. Just take it easy.
9. Try to hear things from the other person's point of view.
10. The harder things get, the more collected I am.
11. It takes two to have conflict, and I'm not going to participate in this.

Do some brainstorming to create phrases you can use in the particularly knotty situations that aggravate you. The statements you devise will probably work best for you. Use them to replace the old automatic, negative self-talk that only adds to your anger, irritability, pain, depression, insecurity, and stress, such as "I'll never be able to handle it," "That guy is a real _____," "I should have done it differently," "I am (a failure/stupid/incompetent)," "I can't bear this any longer," or "I'm so angry right now."

We all talk to ourselves at times. This strategy is designed to increase your awareness of what you are saying to yourself and to keep those inner thoughts as constructive, positive, and health-promoting as possible. What we say to ourselves can help serve as a circuit-breaker for the stress response. If you want to, write the statements that work for you on 3x5 cards, then tape them to your bathroom mirror or to the lamp on your desk. Make them part of your everyday thought processes.

One way to look at this strategy is that you are keeping a guardian at the gate of your mind. Acknowledge what is happening, and seize that instant to engage in solution-oriented thinking and behavior, rather than getting stuck in how you feel about the problem. This shifts you into a position of control and gives you the power to choose the best possible course of action at that moment.

For example, if something goes awry in your life, rather than sinking into a morass of negative self-talk (such as "Oh, no, not another problem, why does this have to happen to me?"), seize the moment to say to yourself, "This is the situation right now . . . what are my options . . . I have the freedom to choose the best solution."

Constructive self-talk is an important part of using your mind as a resource to manage stress more effectively.

"Mental rehearsal" is the second part of strategy number five. Once you're aware of the stressful situations you regularly encounter, or may be dealing with in the near future—and you have developed a list of stressors and arranged them in a hierarchy from least to most stressful—you can begin to use mental rehearsal to minimize that stress and increase the ease with which you incorporate stress management skills into your daily life.

Mental rehearsal is a form of inner blueprinting; you can create new neuronal circuits for healthier behavior patterns by imagining the preferred way in which you'll handle stressful circumstances. The essence of mental rehearsal is to vividly see, hear, and feel yourself successfully responding to and managing the situation at hand, thereby modifying your old behavioral patterns.

To begin mental rehearsal, begin with the first minor stressor on your list. Sit in a comfortable chair and close your eyes. Take a few long, deep breaths and relax your muscles. Picture the situation as vividly as possible, including what you see, hear (say to yourself), and feel. Imagine yourself acting confidently, taking control of, and handling the situation effectively. What are you saying? How are you responding to others? What is your nonverbal behavior? Visualize and feel yourself remaining calm and relaxed.

Keep this image in mind for 20 to 30 seconds. As you do, note any of the early signs of stress in your body—e.g., shallow, arrhythmic breathing or breath-holding, increased heart rate, or increased muscle tension. Use these sensations as signals to relax and implement CIP. In addition, deepen your breathing and relax your muscles, and use some constructive self-talk—a word or phrase that supports you in coping effectively with the situation. For example: "Relax . . . Flow with it . . . What's my best option for dealing with this situation? What attitude will assist me in accomplishing my goal?" If you start to feel tense again, stop, and do CIP to reestablish more positive feelings.

Practice this technique until you are able to mentally rehearse a specific situation twice, each time for about 30 seconds. Once you have accomplished this goal, staying relaxed and calm, without any tension or anxiety, go on to the next, more stressful situation on your list. Over the next week or two, move slowly through the various situations you have listed.

Over time, you'll start noticing that events don't seem nearly as stressful as they once did. When you encounter a situation that used to cause stress, whether it's at work or at home, you'll be much more likely to deal with it effectively and with less stress.

Here are five steps for mental rehearsal:

1. Choose a recent stressful situation that was less than satisfying, in which you intended to but did not apply your CIP and other stress management skills.
2. Take the same scene and rerun it in your mind the way you would have liked to have handled it, using your stress management skills.
3. Observe the first thing you see, hear, or feel that signals you to use your preferred skills. Imagine yourself responding to these cues successfully. Replay this scene a few times in your mind.
4. Actually implement your preferred interaction skills at the first possible opportunity and as frequently as possible.
5. Take a few minutes each day to review your targeted performance objectives and how well you achieved these goals.

By regularly using mental rehearsal, which takes only a few minutes of your time, you can more rapidly, easily, and effectively clean up old habitual patterns and replace them with new, more satisfying ones.

Using CIP and other stress management skills will help you function more of the time in your optimal performance zone and increase your sense of being in control of the stress in your life. In effect, you will be developing a more stress-resistant personality.

VIEW PROBLEMS AS OPPORTUNITIES FOR ENGAGING IN SOLUTION-ORIENTED BEHAVIOR

While CIP is extremely effective for dealing with the stress in your life, there are additional useful strategies available for stress management. CIP can bring your body-mind into balance and reduce the frequency of blood pressure spiking. Frequently, however, in addition to managing stress, the best way to deal with a stressor is to solve, resolve, or eliminate it so it won't keep recurring. For example, if your job is stressful or if your personal interactions are a source of anxiety, it is important to work on these problems constructively.

The Chinese word for crisis is opportunity. Look at problems as opportunities to engage in solution-oriented behavior. This may require some discussion and negotiation with other people involved. It might necessitate delegating responsibility to co-workers so you don't have to carry so much of the load. It may involve changing your behavior—for instance, becoming more assertive in your relationships, asking for what you want, and learning to say no when you repeatedly find yourself taking on too many responsibilities.

Stressors are of different sorts. Some are best managed by letting them pass; others call for active problem-solving in the short- and/or long-term. A HART participant named Mark once said that when problems used to occur in his business, stress would get the better of him and he would "freeze up and nothing would get done." But not anymore. "When an obstacle gets in my way now, I identify it and look for ways to solve it or put it in its place."

Mark identified one of his biggest irritations as the paper flow in his office.

> It made me very uptight and tense. So I decided to get organized and take better control of the flow of paper across my desk. I started putting papers in certain drawers: The top drawer was for the most important papers, those with the highest priority. The middle drawer was of next importance. And in the third drawer, I put low-priority papers—and if I hadn't dealt with them within a week, I would throw them out.

Of course, there are other sources of stress—major and minor—that you can't change rapidly or even with the most creative problem-solving.

They are simply beyond your present control. When these types of situations arise it is useful to recognize them, use your stress management skills, and when appropriate, let go. Dr. Robert Eliot's advice makes sound cardiovascular sense: "Rule No. 1 is, don't sweat the small stuff. Rule No. 2 is, it's all small stuff. And if you can't fight and you can't flee, flow."

Many individuals also benefit from the words by author and philosopher, Reinhold Niebuhr: ". . . grant me the courage to change the things I can, the serenity to accept the things I cannot change, and the wisdom to know the difference."

If you are frequently irritated, angry, anxious, depressed, guilty, bitter or burned out, and are unable to resolve these areas within a reasonable period of time, then it may be advisable to work with a competent therapist.

ACKNOWLEDGING YOUR SUCCESSES

In the weeks ahead, as you implement CIP and the other strategies for effective stress management described in this chapter, warmly acknowledge yourself for your daily successes and even small improvements. Changing behavior is one of the most remarkable human capacities. As you learn to manage the stress in your life, and see the difference it can make in controlling your blood pressure, give yourself credit for having taken control of your own well-being. You deserve to feel good about yourself.

Even after you have achieved proficiency in the basic methods introduced in the biobehavioral core of the HART Program, continue your deep psychophysiological relaxation practice and CIP until you have reached and stabilized your blood pressure at your target goal. Among HART patients, those who continued regular practice experienced ongoing improvements in their blood pressure and reductions in their medication levels. Remember, lower blood pressure minimizes risk and maximizes expected life span. While this is the completion of the biobehavioral component, it is the beginning of a fuller spectrum of non-pharmacological methods that will help you lower your blood pressure and safeguard your cardiovascular health.

SEVEN RECOMMENDATIONS FOR CONTINUING PROGRESS IN THE BIOBEHAVIORAL CORE OF THE HART PROGRAM —

1. Know your goal and how you will achieve it. Set a target blood pressure and vividly imagine engaging in the specific behaviors

useful in achieving and maintaining this goal. See and feel yourself successfully attaining your goal.

2. Until you reach your target blood pressure goal and stabilize it for a few months, continue deep psychophysiological relaxation practice twice daily for fifteen minutes and continue to record your data for one session each day.

3. Continue CIP to incorporate your relaxation skills and stress management skills into daily life.

4. While you are still on blood pressure medication, contact your physician for a medication adjustment at his or her discretion any time your blood pressure remains at or below 140/90 for a two-week period. Provide your doctor with copies of your Daily Blood Pressure log.

5. Once your feedback-assisted relaxation and stress management practice are well-established, it is highly recommended that you incorporate further lifestyle changes, which you will find in Part III of this book. These changes will support you in achieving and maintaining your blood pressure goals and improving your cardiovascular health.

6. If you feel you need or would benefit from additional assistance in implementing your personal nonpharmacologic program to normalize your blood pressure, find a supportive, capable and informed clinician to work with.

7. Regularly monitor your own blood pressure for life. The best protection is prevention. Resume practice of your program skills when your life is particularly stressful or your blood pressure measurements indicate it would be appropriate.

PART III

Lifestyle Changes for Lowering Your Blood Pressure

CHAPTER · 12

Cardiowise Food Selections: Eating for Low Blood Pressure and a Healthy Heart

If you are among the two out of three Americans who do not smoke or drink excessively, your choice of diet can influence your longterm health prospects more than any other action you might take.

> —C. EVERETT KOOP, M.D.,
> Former United States
> Surgeon General

A high intake of complex carbohydrates is definitely associated with a low coronary heart disease mortality, particularly when they are eaten in place of saturated fat.

> —WILLIAM B. KANNEL, M.D.,
> Professor of Medicine,
> Boston University

WE LIVE IN AN ERA of nonfat yogurt, fish oil, and oatbran muffins. More than ever before, people are placing foods and nutrients like these on their dining room tables, with one primary goal in mind: To help them live longer and healthier lives.

If you have high blood pressure, the foods you choose can become a particularly powerful ally in bringing your hypertension under control and protecting you against coronary heart disease. In combination with the other strategies in *The Hart Program* (such as relaxation techniques, stress management strategies, and physical exercise) dietary adjustments have helped many individuals reduce their blood pressure and increase their cardiovascular health.

Food is a primary source of human fuel. The foods we eat, like the thoughts we think and the ways we manage the stresses of life, either contribute to our health or increase our susceptibility to disease. The same basic eating patterns that are conducive to lowering blood pressure can also help prevent heart attacks, strokes, atherosclerosis, arthritis, and cancer.

In these pages, as you learn more about how the foods you select affect your blood pressure, you might discover that you are already nutritionally conscious and are eating a cardiowise diet. On the other hand, if you have been consuming a more typical high-fat, low complex-carbohydrate diet, you may decide to make some significant changes in the way you eat.

There is little controversy surrounding most of the basic nutritional guidelines in this chapter. The majority of these guidelines are in accord with the recommendations of the American Heart Association, the American Cancer Society, and the United States Senate Select Committee on Nutrition and Human Needs. As a result, you may already be familiar with many of them, and hopefully some are already a part of your lifestyle.

This chapter (along with the following two chapters) explains carefully why each nutritional guideline is essential. Briefly, it is worthwhile to take the following dietary recommendations to heart:

1. Reduce the amount of fat you consume.
2. Cut back on dietary cholesterol.
3. Increase your intake of complex carbohydrates and fiber.
4. Reduce your intake of sodium.
5. Make sure your diet contains adequate amounts of calcium, potassium, magnesium, and other minerals and vitamins.
6. Keep your alcohol and caffeine consumption at a moderate level.
7. Normalize your body weight.

If you have high blood pressure, each one of these suggestions can help guide you back toward optimal health. Let's begin to look at them more closely.

REDUCE DIETARY FAT

There is not much good to say about dietary fat, yet thanks to a steady assault of hamburgers, french fries, whole milk, cheese, butter, ice cream, and other common foods, fat accounts for 37 percent of the calories in the typical American diet—a percentage that is much too high for good health. The United States Senate Select Committee on Nutrition and Human Needs recommends that total fat consumption be limited to 30 percent of your total caloric intake; however, if you are at an increased risk because of a high cholesterol level, atherosclerosis, or a history of heart disease, it makes sense to decrease your fat intake even more—to 25, 20, or even 10 percent.

Unfortunately, in foods of animal origin, most calories are from fat. Even in "lean" beef, 40 to 60 percent of its calories are fat. Sirloin steak is about 85 percent fat, and butter and mayonnaise are nearly 100 percent fat!

When former Surgeon General C. Everett Koop issued the government's comprehensive report on nutrition and health in 1988, he singled out the reduction of dietary fat as the nation's most important nutritional priority. Not only does fat contribute to hypertension, it also increases the risk of many other chronic ailments, including coronary heart disease, stroke, diabetes, obesity, and some types of cancer.

How does dietary fat influence blood pressure? A lot of research is going on in this area. Here is one likely scenario: A high-fat diet causes plaque (a buildup of fatty deposits) to form on the inner walls of the arteries. When this happens, the arteries narrow and obstructions develop, forcing a build-up of pressure as the blood travels through the body. Increased pressure, in turn, can cause tearing of the delicate lining of the arteries, which will actually attract more plaque, thus narrowing the arteries and increasing blood pressure even further.

On a diet in which only 10 percent of the calories come from fat, you may be able to slow down the accumulation of arterial plaque, which will retard the progression of your hypertension. There is even some evidence that by significantly reducing your dietary fat intake, you might actually reverse the atherosclerotic process, causing the plaque to decrease in size and allowing the blood to flow easier.

ALL FATS ARE NOT ALIKE

In addition to limiting the total *amount* of fat in your diet, it is useful to begin thinking about the *types* of fats you eat. There are three categories of fats: saturated, monounsaturated, and polyunsaturated. These fats differ from one another in the number of hydrogen atoms in their chemical structure. The worse culprit among them is saturated fat.

Saturated fats are primarily of animal origin, and are generally solid at room temperature. They are contained in foods like butter, hard cheeses, and the marbleized fat on beef. By contrast, both monounsaturated fats and polyunsaturated fats are liquid at room temperature.

However, just because something is labeled as a vegetable oil doesn't necessarily mean it's good for you. In fact, some solid vegetable oils are as bad as those of animal origin. To produce hydrogenated vegetable oils found in some margarines, peanut butter, and other processed foods, manufacturers take perfectly good vegetable oil and alter its hydrogen bonds, creating a saturated fat that is harder than butter.

Coconut oil and palm oil, even though they're in liquid form, aren't any better than the solid variety.

What are the best or healthiest oils? Many liquid fats are better choices. Monounsaturates are the most cardiowise selections, followed by polyunsaturated vegetable oils. Polyunsaturates are a good source of prostaglandins, which are body chemicals essential for proper blood circulation. However, since polyunsaturates can also produce an increase in free radicals in the body—substances that can cause cancer,

THE FATS IN OUR FOODS

Even though foods and oils are generally referred to as saturated, polyunsaturated, or monounsaturated, most foods contain a combination of all three types, with one fat type predominant. Thus a food is considered saturated if it is composed primarily of saturated fats, and polyunsaturated if it is mostly polyunsaturated. The following chart, using figures supplied by the United States Department of Health and Human Services, shows the percentage of total fats of some common foods.*

	Mono-unsaturated fat	Poly-unsaturated fat	Saturated fat
Vegetable oils			
Olive oil	74%	8%	13%
Canola oil	55%	33%	7%
Safflower oil	12%	74%	9%
Sunflower oil	20%	66%	10%
Corn oil	24%	49%	13%
Peanut oil	46%	32%	17%
Palm oil	37%	9%	49%
Coconut oil	6%	2%	86%
**Margarine (soft tub)	47%	31%	18%
**Margarine (stick)	59%	18%	19%
Animal fats			
Beef fat	42%	4%	50%
Chicken fat	45%	21%	30%
Tuna fat (white, packed in water)	26%	37%	27%
Butter fat	29%	4%	62%

**MADE WITH HYDROGENATED SOYBEAN AND COTTONSEED OILS.

especially if they are heated or rancid—polyunsaturates should be used in moderation.

Even though some choices are definitely better than others, fats in general are best when used only sparingly in your personal campaign for good health. In recent years, you may have read that while saturated fats tend to raise your blood cholesterol level, both monounsaturated and polyunsaturated fats do not contribute to plaque formation in the arteries. Now, however, there is some evidence that even unsaturated fats may play a role in the formation of arterial deposits. Thus, while you are wise to shift your selection of fats in the direction of monounsaturates and polyunsaturates, it is a good idea not to use **any** of them in excess. By cutting back on the total amount of fat in your diet, your blood pressure may start to decline.

Consider the findings of a study by American and Finnish researchers who evaluated 57 couples, ages 30 to 50. Some of these volunteers—including both hypertensives and those with normal blood pressure—were placed on a low-fat diet (fats comprising 23 percent of calories), with polyunsaturated fats emphasized over saturated fats and with no changes in salt intake. This diet included foods such as lean meat, low-fat sausage, skim milk, low-fat cheese, vegetables, and margarine high in polyunsaturated fat.

What were the results? After six weeks on the diet, blood pressure dipped from an average of 138/88 to 129/81. The declines were largest in those patients who were hypertensive, with systolic and diastolic decreases averaging 13 mm Hg and 10 mm Hg, respectively.

The Seven Countries Study, a major analysis of the health status of 12,000 people world-wide, took a more general look at the health effects of consuming fat. Researchers found that people in the United States and eastern Finland, whose diets are high in saturated animal fat, had the highest incidence of coronary heart disease. By contrast, the people in Mediterranean countries like Greece and Italy, who rely much more heavily on monounsaturated, plant-derived foods and are more likely to use olive oil than other fats, had many fewer deaths from coronary heart disease. In Japan, where just 10 percent of the dietary calories come from fat, coronary artery disease caused even fewer deaths—**one-tenth** the rate of eastern Finland!

FIGURING OUT FOOD FAT CONTENT

Although it is best to rely on fresh, unprocessed foods whenever possible, everyone invariably puts some packaged items into his or her shopping cart. If you're not a careful label-reader, you can send your fat intake soaring by making too many inappropriate choices.

When you pick up a food item, look for the *Nutrition Information* section on the label. This section tells you the amounts of calories, protein, carbohydrates, and fat per serving. It's a lot of data—but you will need even **more** information to make a wise decision. While the label might tell you that the food item has 240 calories and 8 grams of fat per serving, you still need to calculate the **percentage** of the calories that come from fat. If it turns out to be 20 percent, then you've made a good choice; if it's 40 percent, you are better off looking for another product.

With food labeling laws demanding ever more detailed product information, it will eventually become easier to determine the percentage of calories from fat in processed foods without carrying your calculator to the supermarket. In the meantime, here's how to figure out a particular item's fat content:

1. Multiply the number of grams of fat in each serving by 9. Since every gram of fat contains 9 calories, the answer will correspond to the number of **fat** calories per serving. In the example above, you would multiply 9 calories by 8 grams ($9 \times 8 = 72$).
2. Next, take this answer and divide it by the total number of calories in the serving. In our example, that would mean dividing 72 calories by 240 ($72 \div 240 = .30$).
3. Then take that number and multiply it by 100 by moving the decimal point two digits to the right, thus converting it to a percentage ($.30 \div 100 = 30$ percent).
4. In this example, the food item has a fat content of 30 percent. Not bad. You might be able to do even better, however, by comparing products.

REDUCE DIETARY CHOLESTEROL

As you reduce the fat in your diet—by cutting back on foods like red meat, high-fat cheese and whole milk—another important nutritional change will almost automatically occur at the same time—namely, a reduction in the amount of cholesterol you consume. Dietary cholesterol is yet another potential troublemaker in the hypertension-cardiovascular disease story, so the less of it you eat, the better.

You won't find dietary cholesterol in unprocessed, high complex carbohydrate plant foods, including vegetables, fruits, cereals, and beans; rather, it is present only in foods of animal origin, including beef, lamb, pork, poultry, organ meats (liver, sweetbreads), and egg yolks.

Along with saturated fats, dietary cholesterol can raise your blood cholesterol level to dangerous heights, i.e. increasing your risk of developing coronary heart disease and hypertension.

Low-fat foods are usually low in cholesterol as well, but there are some exceptions:

1. **Eggs.** Although the average egg is low in saturated fat, it is very high in cholesterol (about 270 mg)—the yolk is largely the cause. The white of the egg, however, is high in protein and low in cholesterol. Limit the number of egg yolks in your diet. If you want scrambled eggs for breakfast, use two to three egg whites for each yolk; or, if you cook other things with eggs, use just the whites or egg substitutes.

2. **Shellfish.** Many kinds of shellfish, such as shrimp, lobster, oysters, and clams, are high in cholesterol, even though they are low in fat. Although it is fine to substitute these shellfish for other types of seafood once in a while, it's best not to make it a habit, particularly if your blood cholesterol level is high. However, other types of shellfish from the mollusk family—such as scallops and mussels—are moderately low in cholesterol and calories.

YOUR CHOLESTEROL COUNT

It may sound surprising, but everyone needs some cholesterol. In fact, the liver even manufactures a modest amount of this white, waxy substance. The body uses cholesterol to build cell walls and to manufacture hormones and other vital substances.

If you are like many people, however, you have an excess of cholesterol in your body, largely because you eat too much saturated fat and dietary cholesterol. This can be dangerous. Researchers have concluded that **the higher your cholesterol reading, the greater your risk of developing coronary heart disease.** According to one study, the likelihood of dying from heart disease is 72 percent greater if your total blood cholesterol level is 220 mg/dl (milligrams per deciliter) or higher, rather than below 220 mg/dl. Since the average cholesterol reading of people who suffer heart attacks is about 220, some doctors are still telling their patients that a cholesterol of 220 is "normal," giving them a false sense of security rather than motivating them to take expedient, preventive action to lower their risk of cardiovascular disease.

CHOLESTEROL GUIDELINES

In 1987, the National Cholesterol Education Program's expert panel convened to create guidelines to help the public and physicians better understand cholesterol and the risks associated with it. After evaluating the growing body of research on the subject, they created the following cholesterol guidelines:

If your cholesterol is less than 200 mg/dl, you have a *desirable* blood cholesterol level.
If your cholesterol reading falls between 200 mg/dl and 239 mg/dl, your level is *borderline high.*
If your cholesterol level is greater than 240 mg/dl, you have a *high cholesterol count.*

Anyone with a blood cholesterol level of 200 or more would be wise to work on lowering it. A cholesterol count below 200 provides added protection against heart attacks and strokes, while **a level of 150 is considered optimal for longevity.**

YOUR CHOLESTEROL RATIO

As the first step in determining whether you need to reduce your cholesterol, have your cholesterol level checked. At that time, ask your doctor about your cholesterol *subfractions*—that is, have him or her determine your high-density lipoprotein (HDL) and low-density lipoprotein (LDL) readings. As important as your total cholesterol level is, it's not the whole story. Cholesterol travels through your bloodstream joined to either of these two major types of protein. While one of them—the LDL or "bad" cholesterol—promotes the formation of plaque on your arterial walls, the other—HDL or "good" cholesterol—works the opposite way, functioning as a scavenger that removes fats from the arteries and carries them to the liver to be excreted from the body. For that reason, **a cardiowise goal is to reduce your LDL level while keeping your HDL count high.**

How will your doctor determine whether your LDL and HDL levels are safe? Doctors usually look at the ratio of your total cholesterol to your HDL level. For example:

If your total cholesterol = 220 mg/dl
And your HDL cholesterol = 50 mg/dl
Your ratio = 220/50 or 4.4.

In the United States, the average cholesterol ratio is 4.5 for males and 4.0 for females. You can do even better by setting and reaching the goal of a ratio no higher than 3.5.

Let's examine the importance of this ratio. Assume that you and your spouse both have total blood cholesterol levels of 210. However, your protective HDL level is 60 (for a ratio of 3.5) and your spouse's is 45 (a ratio of 4.7). Since the lower the ratio, the better, you have less to worry about when it comes to coronary heart disease.

A final point: If you have high blood pressure, it is particularly important for you to lower your total blood cholesterol level and your cholesterol ratio. Researchers now know that when it comes to heart attacks, the presence of both hypertension and high blood cholesterol increases your risk of having a heart attack more than either factor alone. So make the dietary changes necessary to get your blood cholesterol count under control.

THE DIETARY BENEFITS OF FISH

The life of a Greenland Eskimo may not sound particularly appealing. Nonetheless, there are some real health advantages to their chilly existence; most notably, Eskimos have low blood pressure and a low incidence of heart disease.

For years, researchers have been trying to figure out why Eskimos are nearly free of heart attacks. A diet rich in fish may be the answer. Eskimos consume over 14 ounces of fish, whale, and seal meat a day, a diet that seems to provide considerable cardiovascular protection.

Fortunately, studies also suggest that you can protect your own heart even by eating much smaller amounts of fish. Dutch scientist Daan Kromhout found that men who consumed an ounce of fish or more a day over a 20-year span were two and a half times less likely to die of heart disease than men who ate no fish.

What is responsible for this positive effect of fish upon the cardiovascular system? Several studies have suggested that fish oils—particularly, a polyunsaturated fish oil called omega-3—may play a role. Among other benefits, omega-3 apparently helps reduce blood pressure and cholesterol, although as yet, the mechanism responsible for this decline is unknown.

What follows are the findings of two recent studies:

1. At Vanderbilt University, researchers monitored 32 men with mild hypertension. Only some of them were given fish oil supplements. The men who received a high dose (50 ml) of fish oil each day experienced an average decline of 6.5 mm Hg in their systolic blood pressure over four weeks, along with a 4.4 mm Hg reduction in their diastolic reading. A lower dose (10 ml) of fish oil per day produced no significant changes in blood pressure measurements.
2. A British study at Chelmsford and Essex Hospital found positive effects on blood pressure from fish-oil supplementation. After six weeks of treatment, sixteen men and women (average age, 55) experienced average reductions in blood pressure from 160/94 to 151/92.5 mm Hg.

The news about fish oil, then, is encouraging. However, that doesn't mean that you can continue to eat steak, eggs, and other high-fat, high-cholesterol dishes, and then rely on an occasional fish dish to come to your rescue. As for fish oil capsules, the Food and Drug Administration halted their sale in 1990, pointing to their unproven safety and questionable effect on coronary heart disease.

Even before the FDA's ban on fish oil pills, most responsible nutritionists were convinced that people were better off obtaining their fish oil by eating fish itself. This is still the healthiest approach. The types of fish that are particularly rich in omega-3 include salmon, pompano, chinook, herring, mackerel, bonito, trout, albacore, shad, and bluefish.

There are other factors to keep in mind when choosing and preparing fish: It's best to select deep water, ocean, or farm-raised fish over lake or river fish, in order to minimize possible pollutants in your diet. When you're looking for alternatives to fresh fish, frozen fish is the next best option. If you choose canned fish instead, look for water-packed over oil-packed varieties.

THE DIETARY BENEFITS OF COMPLEX CARBOHYDRATES

A high complex-carbohydrate diet is an important key to a healthy heart and cardiovascular system. Complex carbohydrates, found in vegetables, fruits, and grains, are longevity foods. As you raise the percentage of these foods in your diet, your chances for a longer and healthier life increase as well.

Here are the facts: A diet rich in complex carbohydrates directly combats three major risk factors for heart disease: high blood pressure, high blood cholesterol levels, and obesity. In countries with a low prevalence of atherosclerosis, people obtain about 60 to 80 percent of their calories from carbohydrates, particularly complex carbohydrates. However, the majority of Americans, like many populations in the Western world, don't do as well. About 40 to 45 percent of our calories come from carbohydrates, and as many as one-half of these come from refined sugars. In turn, we have a high rate of atherosclerosis and high blood pressure.

As a species, we are physiologically designed to eat a diet high in complex carbohydrates and low in fat. Evolutionarily, our teeth and mouth are more structured for eating vegetables, fruits, and grains. So is our lengthy intestinal tract and the amount of hydrochloric acid (useful in digesting a high-meat diet) produced. (By contrast, meat-eating animals have canine teeth and short intestinal tracts, and produce about 20 percent more hydrochloric acid than we do.) Unfortunately, in modern times, the typical diet in Western nations has emphasized animal protein and dairy products.

Population studies have repeatedly demonstrated the benefits of eating lots of complex carbohydrates. One of the most impressive of these is the ten-year-long Zutphen Study, which concluded that the death rate from coronary heart disease was four times greater in individuals who consumed the lowest amounts of complex carbohydrates. **A review of dietary patterns in more than two dozen cultures has shown that those consuming the highest levels of complex carbohydrates and least amounts of fats had the lowest incidence of heart disease. Most strikingly, when the customary diet included just 10 to 12 percent of its calories from fat, heart disease was almost nonexistent.**

EATING PATTERNS IN DIFFERENT CULTURES

As the table below illustrates,* Western societies—in which cardiovascular disease is most prevalent—consume only about half the carbohydrates and more than four times the fat of Oriental and developing nations.

	Carbohydrates %	Fat %	Protein%
Western	45	43	12
Oriental	80	10	10
Developing	80	10	10

* ADAPTED FROM JULIAN M. WHITAKER, *REVERSING HEART DISEASE*.

Research like this indicates that the most cardiowise diet centers around complex carbohydrates. Complex carbohydrates offer a number of advantages:

They are the primary source of energy in the diet, and are excellent endurance foods, providing the body with sustainable fuel.

They are lower in calories than fat (containing less than half the number of calories per ounce), and thus are particularly good choices if you are watching your weight.

They are rich in vitamins and minerals that may help lower blood pressure and protect against cardiovascular disease. (The next chapter presents evidence suggesting that calcium, potassium, magnesium, vitamin C, and other nutrients may help normalize blood pressure. Complex carbohydrates are rich sources of these vitamins and minerals.)

They are the preferred food for stress management, providing added resilience and a buffer in dealing with day-to-day stress. More than any other food category, complex carbohydrates have a calming effect. In one study, researchers examined the effects of a high-carbohydrate meal as opposed to a high-protein meal on 184 healthy adults. After consuming the high-carbohydrate meal, male subjects reported feeling calmer, while women tended to feel sleepier. The high-protein meals, however, increased tension levels in many subjects, especially those ages 40 or older. For this reason, complex carbohydrates are often recommended for people under stress who would like to feel more relaxed, or for individuals who want to sleep more deeply.

Researchers have discovered that the intake of carbohydrates leads to significant changes in brain chemistry, most noticeably a rise in serotonin, a chemical which can induce feelings of calm and satisfaction, and help alleviate anxiety. This serotonin increase is the direct result of elevated levels of tryptophan (an amino acid) that accompany carbohydrate intake.

Eating a dinner high in complex carbohydrates and low in protein and fat can help promote a deep and restful night's sleep. Meals high in protein—which contribute to alertness—are good choices earlier in the day when your work is ahead of you.

Complex carbohydrates can be good sources of fiber, which has important dietary advantages that deserve further explanation.

THE BENEFITS OF DIETARY FIBER

Sometimes called *roughage*, dietary fiber is a component of plant material, and is necessary for good digestion and elimination. By drawing water into the digestive system, fiber softens the stool and thus helps minimize constipation. Even more important, fiber may help prevent certain kinds of cancer, particularly colon cancer, by speeding up the passage of cancer-causing substances through the digestive tract. Fiber can also reduce the incidence of hemorrhoids, diverticulosis, and other common gastrointestinal problems.

Fiber's positive effects on hypertension are just as impressive. Several studies have shown that people with a high intake of dietary fiber have substantially reduced their blood pressure: The consumption of 24 to 45 grams of fiber per day can cut blood pressure an average of 3 to 10 mm Hg.

In a British study, seventeen healthy volunteers were monitored for three weeks while eating their usual low-fiber diet (16.2 grams of fiber per day). Then their fiber intake was increased to 24.5 grams per day during the ensuing four weeks. On the higher-fiber diets, systolic blood pressure dropped 3.2 percent, while diastolic values fell 4.7 percent.

Research by Dr. James Anderson at the University of Kentucky College of Medicine evaluated the blood pressure readings of 12 nonobese, diabetic men. For one week, these men were fed a traditional diet that included 20 grams of fiber per day; on this so-called control diet, carbohydrates provided 43 percent of calories. Then these men switched to a high-fiber, high-carbohydrate diet, which included 65 grams of fiber per day. Carbohydrates on this followup diet provided 70 percent of calories.

After fourteen days, blood pressures were measured. The results: Every patient had lower blood pressure values, with average declines of 10 percent, and slightly greater decreases in those men who had hypertension. At the same time, these diabetics were able to reduce their insulin doses by 73 percent on the high-fiber regimen; their cholesterol readings plummeted, too, from an average of 217 mg/dl to 161 mg/dl.

Fiber can also help reduce your blood cholesterol level by adhering to the fats in your diet and transporting them out of the body.

Yet despite these proven benefits, many people have not gotten the message. In the United States, we consume about one-third less fiber than our own ancestors did at the turn of the twentieth century. We need to play catch-up. You will get the greatest overall benefit from this program if you add lots of fiber to your diet by making commonly available foods like vegetables, fruits, legumes, and whole-grain breads and cereals an integral part of your meals. Certain types of fiber—the water-soluble fibers—are particularly effective in reducing blood cholesterol levels. Good sources of soluble fiber include oat bran, rice bran, barley, fruit, and dried beans.

HOW MUCH FIBER IS IN YOUR FOOD?

	High-Fiber Foods	Low-Fiber Foods
Vegetables	Vegetables that are raw, lightly-boiled, steamed, or stir-fried	Vegetables that are over-cooked
Fruit	Fresh fruits, such as apples, pears, plums, bananas, apricots	Cooked, canned fruit; fruit juice
Breads	Whole-grain bread	Breads made of refined flour (white, sourdough, and French bread)
Other foods	Legumes, brown rice, wild rice, whole wheat, popcorn	Refined flour

To maximize the benefits of fiber in the diet, eat foods as close to their natural state as possible. For instance, as healthful as a glass of orange juice is, eating a whole orange is even better. Choose whole wheat bread or rye, not white bread. Eat many of your vegetables raw, including cucumbers, green peppers, tomatoes, carrots, broccoli, and cauliflower. Also, eat the skins of vegetables and fruits like potatoes and apples after thoroughly washing them to remove pesticides.

Does fiber have a downside? In **extremely** high amounts, fiber might bind to certain minerals (such as calcium, iron, magnesium, copper, zinc) and carry them out of the body instead of allowing them to be absorbed into the bloodstream. So while you can safely eat large amounts of dietary fiber, it is still best not to go overboard.

REDUCE REFINED CARBOHYDRATES AND SUGARS

As good as complex carbohydrates are for you, it is wise to limit refined carbohydrates—such as foods made with white, refined flour and sugar—in your diet. White starches—like white breads, pastas, white rice, and snack foods—are refined carbohydrates, and belong in the same "less desirable" category.

Even though sugar is about eight times more refined than white starch, the white starches can still contribute to disease susceptibility because fiber and valuable nutrients have been extracted from what started out as wholesome food. Products made with white, refined flour are a source of "devitaminized," non-nutritious, empty calories. Don't be led astray by the "enriched" label on processed foods; little real nutrition has been put back in compared to what has been taken out. By contrast, breads made from whole grains truly are the staff of life. Sugar itself is brimming with calories, yet it has only minimal nutrients. Nevertheless, we are a nation seemingly obsessed with it, almost to the point of addiction to soft drinks, cookies and cakes. Sugar is also hidden in foods ranging from frozen dinners to salad dressings. No wonder the average American eats a startling one-third of a pound of sugar every day.

There have been only a few studies on the effects of sugar on blood pressure. They show that sugar may increase blood pressure while decreasing the excretion of sodium. In one of these studies, volunteers were given up to 200 mg of sucrose a day for five weeks; their blood pressure increased an average of 5 mm Hg.

In animal research, the blood pressure of spider monkeys rose significantly higher when the monkeys were given sucrose along with sodium chloride, rather than just sodium chloride alone. Some special strains of hypertensive rats showed significant increases in their blood pressure readings when they were fed sugar and salt. Their blood pressure declined when sugar was removed from the diet, but not when salt was eliminated.

Sugar is also a mood-altering food. Even though it can certainly create a "sugar high" in the short run, many individuals soon experience corresponding declines in energy and feelings of well-being as the body dumps increased insulin into the bloodstream and causes a plunge in glucose that can result in fatigue, irritability, and anxiety. When this occurs, people often feel the urge to reach for more sugar-rich products to combat the "post-sugar blues," which only perpetuates this less-than-healthy eating cycle.

Different types of sweeteners can have very different effects on your blood sugar level. Pure glucose is a "fast releaser," ranking high (at the 100 percent level) on the *glycemic index,* a measurement of the effect of food components upon blood sugar. It is a poor choice for people trying to control their blood sugar. Honey is somewhat lower (87 percent on the glycemic index) and sucrose is even better (59 percent). Yet fructose, (fruit sugar), with an even lower glycemic index (20 percent), is clearly the best choice; fructose sweetens food but is less likely to cause a hypoglycemic reaction: low blood sugar, characterized by fatigue, weakness, shakiness, and headaches.

A benefit of filling up on complex carbohydrates like whole grains, fruits, and vegetables is that there won't be much room on your plate for sugar-laden items. So instead of eating sugar-rich, high-cholesterol desserts made with white refined flour, emphasize fresh fruit or baked goods made with whole grains and sweetened with fresh fruit or fresh fruit concentrates. As a general principle, the more whole the food you use as a source of sweetener, the better; thus, a chopped-up natural fruit is preferred over granulated fructose.

WHAT ABOUT GARLIC AND ONIONS?

Do garlic and onions contribute to cardiovascular health? There is still a lot of debate on this question. Even so, a number of studies indicate that large amounts of garlic (3 gloves or 10 grams per day) may lower blood cholesterol levels, raise HDL ("good") cholesterol values, reduce triglycerides (fatty substances in the blood), and even lower blood pressure. Although the evidence is still not conclusive, here is some of what we know:

A dietary study was conducted in a community in India in which subjects were classified according to how often they ate garlic and onions—either frequently, occasionally, or not at all. Blood tests revealed that both cholesterol and triglyceride levels were strikingly lower among the "frequent" consumers of these foods. For instance, while cholesterol levels averaged 159 mg/dl for those in the "frequent" group, they were 172 for the "occasional" users and 208 for the "nonusers."

In another study, 20 healthy volunteers were followed for six months, during which time they consumed 15 mg per day of essential oil of garlic, equal to about 30 grams of whole garlic. The protective HDL levels rose 40 percent in these individuals, while total cholesterol declined 16 percent. A separate study of 62 coronary heart disease patients found a 23 percent decrease in blood cholesterol (compared to control subjects) after 10 months on 15 mg of oil of garlic per day.

In 1987, researchers reported the first double-blind, controlled human study of garlic. Twenty healthy subjects were given 18 mg per day of garlic oil. After a month, their blood cholesterol level dropped 16 percent, while their HDL values increased 23 percent. At the same time, their mean blood pressure declined significantly, from an average of 94 mm Hg to 88 mm Hg.

Garlic and onions may someday play a routine role in cardiovascular care. For now, if you find this food tasty, enjoy it with the knowledge that you might also be helping your heart and blood pressure.

WHAT ABOUT CAFFEINE?

Caffeine is a nervous system stimulant, found in cola, cocoa, coffee, and tea. It can help keep you awake and alert, which might seem particularly attractive on groggy mornings or during 4:00 lows and late-night work marathons. But the caffeine in coffee can also trigger an alarm reaction, increasing nervousness and anxiety and interfering with sleep even when you want to rest.

Caffeine also has a short-term ability to raise your blood pressure. Within fifteen minutes after drinking two to three cups of brewed coffee, for instance, your blood pressure may rise 5 to 15 mm Hg, particularly if you are not a regular coffee drinker. However, it will remain at that higher level for only a short time, perhaps just a couple hours.

In one study with ten volunteers, blood pressure values rose in response to caffeine consumption; but after several days, these measurements remained at their original levels during the subsequent four weeks, even though these subjects continued to drink coffee. So while caffeine may elevate your blood pressure, your body will rapidly build up a tolerance to it.

If you do regularly drink beverages with caffeine, learn when to cut back or substitute decaffeinated alternatives. Water-extract decaffeinated coffees are widely available, which may be a better option than chemical-extract decaf because of the potential cancer-causing properties of the latter. One option is to mix fresh ground, water-extract decaf coffee with some caffeinated coffee. Decaf teas and even decaf soft drinks are also readily available.

WHAT ABOUT ALCOHOL?

Alcohol consumption is on the rise in the United States, and its connection to hypertension has become stronger with each new study. For instance, a large study in Sydney, Australia, which monitored 20,920 people, concluded that blood pressure readings rose with increases in alcohol intake. Similar conclusions were reached by investigators in the 10,000-person Intersalt study. Australian researchers have estimated that 10 percent of hypertension in men and 1 percent in women are caused by alcohol use.

Now for the good news: If you stop drinking or significantly curtail your alcohol intake, this can have a rapid and positive effect on your blood pressure. In one study, researchers inquired about the drinking habits of patients as they were admitted to a hospital. More than half of the individuals who typically consumed over three ounces of alcohol a day had high blood pressure. However, by the time they were discharged from the hospital—where their regular drinking habits had been interrupted—less than one-tenth of them still had hypertension.

There's one ironic twist to the alcohol story: a moderate intake— perhaps a drink or two a day—may actually boost your HDL or "good" cholesterol level, which would be an important benefit. Even so, this isn't the complete picture. There is actually more than one type of HDL cholesterol, and the kind increased by alcohol may **not** be the type that provides protection for the heart. For that reason, if you're a non-drinker, don't begin consuming alcohol just because it might raise your HDL level. We need more information before making recommendations like that.

If you already drink, do so in moderation. Standard guidelines suggest limiting your consumption to no more than one to two ounces of alcohol per day. That's the equivalent of 12 to 24 ounces of beer, 4 to 8 ounces of wine, or 1 to 2 ounces of 100 proof distilled spirits.

YOUR SENSIBLE CARDIOWISE EATING PLAN

How can you select a cardiowise eating plan? If you have high blood pressure—with a normal cholesterol level and no other cardiovascular problems or family history of heart disease—aim for a diet composed of about 60 percent complex carbohydrates, 25 percent fat, and 15 percent protein. However, if your cholesterol level is high, or if you have had a heart attack or have a family history of heart disease, you may be wise to lower your fat intake even further—to as little as 10 percent of your caloric intake.

Of course, it is not realistic to expect you to spend your time constantly calculating exactly how much you are consuming in each food category. For this reason, it will be helpful to consult the food selection charts at the end of this chapter. These charts divide food into four groups—from the healthiest (Group 1) to the least healthy (Group 4). Make as many of your food choices as possible from Group 1. You should eat foods in Groups 2 and 3 only in moderation, and consume foods in Group 4 sparingly.

For a diet high in complex carbohydrates, select **fresh** vegetables, fruits, and **unrefined** grains whenever possible. Also prepare your foods in a healthy way. This means cutting off all skin and visible fat from poultry and meat before cooking; preparing poultry, fish, and meat by broiling, baking, poaching, and roasting, and staying away from deep frying. For vegetables, steam or stir-fry them for several minutes. This is the best way to preserve most of their vitamins. Rather than cooking with butter, use monounsaturated oils such as olive and canola, or nonfat yogurt, instead.

With combinations of grains, legumes, low-fat dairy products, and seeds you can consume high-quality proteins equal to the protein in animal meat, but with much lower fat content. According to Frances Moore Lappe, author of *Diet for a Small Planet*, "The three most common complementary protein combinations are (1) grains (e.g., rice, corn, wheat, barley) with legumes; (2) any grain plus a milk product;

and (3) seeds (sesame, sunflower) with legumes (peas, beans, lentils)."

Keep lower-fat, animal protein consumption to about three to four ounces per serving, but no more than six to eight ounces per day. This includes skinned chicken, turkey, or fish. Limit red meat consumption to leaner cuts, no more than twice a week, and to small portions. Remember to trim the visible fat before cooking. If from time to time, you do eat foods high in fat, whether entrees or desserts, limit portion sizes. And if you are restricting your fat intake to closer to 10 percent for health reasons, think of and use all animal meats as condiments, and concentrate on meeting your protein needs by combining whole grains, legumes, and non-fat dairy products.

If you don't have a high blood cholesterol level, restrictions on dairy products are less critical if they are **nonfat,** but minimize those dairy products made with whole milk and higher-fat (and often high-sodium) cheeses. If you are at your preferred weight, there is no need to limit the amount of whole grains, fruits and vegetables you eat—unless you are cooking with butter, salt, and sugar. In that case, you need to treat them like any high-fat, salt-, or sugar-laden food, and eat them sparingly.

EATING OUT

When eating out, it takes extra creativity and the willingness to ask for what you want in order to keep control over the way your food is prepared. In today's health-conscious world, most chefs are used to food-preparation requests from patrons. You should try to choose restaurants that willingly accommodate your special dietary needs and cook food to order. Be politely assertive. Ask questions about how the food is prepared. If need be, let your waiter or waitress know you are under medical care and that your requests are doctor's orders.

You can order vegetable dishes freely, but make certain they're not cooked in large amounts of oil or sautéed in butter. Your meals should **not** be prepared with salt, Monosodium Glutamate (MSG), or soy sauce. Also, request that sauces, gravies, or dressings be omitted or served on the side. For your salad dressing, lemon wedges and vinegar-and-oil are good choices, and if you like, fresh sliced onions. Also order your potatoes baked and dry.

THE EFFECTS OF A CARDIOWISE EATING PLAN

A 1990 study helps put cardiowise nutritional programs in perspective and shows how powerful overall lifestyle changes can be. Dr. Dean

Ornish of the University of California at San Francisco put his heart-disease patients (ages 35 to 75) on a very strict diet, consisting of a near-vegetarian program in which about 10 percent of the calories came from fat. Patients could drink a modest amount of alcohol (up to two ounces a day), but no caffeine or cigarettes. They practiced relaxation and meditation techniques, and devoted 30 minutes three times a week to exercise, most often walking.

After one year, the chest pain in most of these patients was gone. Most strikingly, in 82 percent of the individuals, **the blockages in their arteries had been significantly reduced and reversed.** By contrast, another group of patients who received traditional care, and who consumed about 30 percent of their calories in dietary fat, experienced a worsening of their chest pain and a progression of their heart disease.

The next chapter discusses how minerals and vitamins in your diet may have the potential to raise or lower your blood pressure.

FOUR FOOD GROUPS

Make as many of your food choices as possible from Group 1. Eat foods from Groups 2 and 3 in moderation and from Group 4 sparingly.

Group 1

Vegetables

artichokes	kale
asparagus	leeks
bamboo shoots	lettuce (all varieties)
beets	mushrooms
bell peppers	mustard greens
broccoli	okra
Brussels sprouts	onions
cabbage (all varieties)	parsley
carrots	potatoes
cauliflower	pumpkin
celery	radishes
chili peppers	rutabagas
corn	scallions
cucumbers	shallots
eggplant	snap beans
endive	sorrel
escarole	spinach
garlic	sprouts (all types)
ginger root	squash (all types)

sweet potatoes
tomatoes
turnips and greens

watercress
yams
zucchini

Fruit

Nearly all fresh fruit, including:

apples
apricots
bananas
blackberries
blueberries
boysenberries
cantaloupe
casaba melon
cherries
cranberries
currents
dates
figs
grapefruit
grapes
guava
honeydew melon
kiwi fruit
kumquats

lemons
limes
mangoes
nectarines
oranges
papayas
peaches
pears
pineapples
plums
pomegranates
prunes
quinces
raisins
raspberries
strawberries
tangerines
watermelons

Grains

All whole grains, such as:

barley
bread
buckwheat
bulgur
cereals (granola free of sugar
  or coconut, shredded wheat,
  oatmeal)
corn, corn meal, corn flour,
  popcorn
crackers (whole wheat, rice)

millet
oats
rice (wild, whole grain)
rye
sorghum grain
soybeans
tortillas
wheat (whole grain, rolled,
  cracked, germ, bran)

Legumes

All cooked legumes, such as:

azuki beans
black beans

black-eyed beans
brown-eyed peas

chick-peas (garbanzos)
Great Northern beans
kidney beans
lentils
navy beans
peas
pinto beans

red Mexican beans
soybeans
soy flour
soy milk
split peas
sprouts
tofu

Miscellaneous

egg whites

brewer's yeast

Group 2

Fish

abalone
albacore
bass
bonito
bluefish
catfish
chinook
cod
flounder
grouper
haddock
halibut
herring
mackerel

mussels
perch
pollack
pompano
salmon
shad
snapper
sole
sturgeon
swordfish
trout
tuna
white fish

Dairy

nonfat plain yogurt

skim milk

Oils

olive oil

canola oil

Miscellaneous

fructose

unsweetened fruit concentrate
(for sweeteners)

Group 3

Meat

chicken
turkey

(bake or broil, with skin and
fat removed before cooking;
white meat is lower in fat)

Seafood

crab
eel
sardines

scallops
shrimp (on occasion)

Oils

corn oil
corn oil margarine (stick,
  unhydrogenated)

safflower oil
sesame oil
soy margarine

Dairy

low-fat skim cheeses (hoop,
  mozzarella, farmer, un-
  creamed cottage cheese)

skim milk
low-fat yogurt

Miscellaneous

honey

Group 4

Whole Milk Dairy Products

cream
cream cheese
whole milk

whole milk cheeses
whole milk yogurt

Meat

all beef products (choose lean-
  est cuts, remove fat before
  cooking)

all pork products

Poultry

fried chicken, with skin

Fruit

avocado

coconut

Miscellaneous

egg yolks
fried foods
high-salt foods

pure maple syrup
white refined & brown sugar

CHAPTER 13

Sizing Up Vitamins and Minerals: What Helps, What Hurts?

Dietary potassium, calcium, magnesium . . . are other aspects of nutrition that may have a significant influence on blood pressure, and these are now under active research.

—ROSE STAMLER, M.A.
JEREMIAH STAMLER, M.D.,
Northwestern University
Medical School

MORE THAN ANY OTHER MINERAL, sodium—a component of salt—has been blamed for increases in blood pressure. In this chapter, we will not only discuss the evidence linking sodium and hypertension, but also the role that other minerals and vitamins may play in lowering your blood pressure and protecting your cardiovascular health.

For some of these vitamins and minerals—particularly sodium—the evidence is quite persuasive regarding the effect they have on hypertension. With calcium, potassium, magnesium, and others, there is not yet a consensus on whether they are important for normalizing blood pressure. However, even though the evidence may not yet be conclusive, the results of some studies and nutritional surveys are sufficiently promising to indicate that some of these minerals and vitamins may someday become a standard part of the nonpharmacological antihypertensive arsenal. Until then, if you are committed to using nondrug approaches to normalizing your blood pressure, the following information on the relationship of minerals and vitamins to blood pressure and cardiovascular health can assist you in making informed, nutritional selections that may help you control your hypertension and protect your overall well-being.

SHAKE THE SALT HABIT

In a respected medical textbook, Dr. Norman Kaplan used the following (somewhat simplified) scenario to portray how high blood pressure may develop in some individuals. He described a young man whose parents both had hypertension, but whose own blood pressure was normal early in life. This young man consumed the average American diet, had an active lifestyle, and his weight was normal. Still, with the passage of time, his blood pressure began to increase. Due to heredity, his body was apparently not excreting the excess sodium in his diet. Most of the sodium ended up in his blood plasma and bodily fluids, which in turn caused water to be retained—boosting the volume of the blood and fluids. The ultimate result: higher blood pressure.

Simultaneously, sodium was also settling into the muscles within this man's arterial walls, setting off a chain of chemical processes that made his blood pressure rise even higher. Before long, this patient's doctor had diagnosed him as having hypertension—apparently all because of his sodium intake.

Before going further, let's define some terms. Although *sodium* and *salt* are often used interchangeably, there are differences between them. Sodium is a mineral that is a component of salt. The white crystal we call salt, or sodium chloride, is made up of about 40 percent sodium; the remainder is chloride.

Just like cholesterol, sodium is a substance that our bodies can't do without, although we could get by quite well with much less of it. In very small amounts, this mineral is necessary for nerve impulses to be properly transmitted, and for maintaining proper blood volume within the blood vessels. Sodium helps muscle tissue contract, and keeps various fluids in the body at appropriate levels.

According to researchers at Northwestern University however, a high sodium diet may prime your brain to be extra sensitive to stress. Specifically, salt increases the number of brain-cell receptors for norepinephrine (or adrenalin), the hormone that prepares the body to fight or flee in response to perceived threats. When signaled by the brain, norepinephrine terminals throughout the body transmit a message to speed up the heart rate and constrict blood vessels, which also raises blood pressure. Thus, the more brain cell receptors that receive norepinephrine, the more susceptible you may be to stress.

In earlier eras, the salt shaker was not the temptation it is today. Salt was actually a scarce commodity throughout much of recorded history, with some societies actually going to war over it. Today, salt is second only to sugar as the most popular food additive in the United States. If you're like the average American, you consume many times the amount of salt your body needs. In an update of its nutritional recommendations, the National Research Council recently advised that the average adult could get along on just 500 mg of salt, or about one-fourth of a teaspoon a day. "Although no optimal range of salt intake has been established, **there is no known advantage in consuming large amounts**

of sodium and clear disadvantages for those susceptible to hypertension," the council proclaimed.

If your doctor has warned you to cut back on your sodium intake, you need to do much more than conceal the salt shaker. About two-thirds of the sodium we consume is hidden in an array of mostly prepackaged (boxed, canned, frozen) or precooked foods, including sandwich meats, snacks, canned soups, sauces, cereals, margarine, pudding, canned vegetables, and condiments. For this reason, it is important to become an avid label-reader and to familiarize yourself with the sodium content of common foods. Who would think, for example, that a typical all-beef hot dog would contain more than 600 mg of sodium, not to mention that 80 percent of its 145 calories are fat calories? Soft drinks contain sodium, as does baking soda, baking powder, and even medications such as antacids.

SODIUM CONTENT OF COMMON FOODS _____

	mg of sodium
asparagus, fresh (1/2 cup)	1
tomato, fresh (1/2 cup)	4
potato, baked (1 medium)	4
peas, fresh (1/2 cup)	15
bran flakes (3/4 cup)	156
peas, canned (1/2 cup)	200
asparagus, canned (1/2 cup)	235
tomato juice (1/2 cup)	243
buttermilk (low fat, 1 cup)	319
potato au gratin (1/2 cup)	529
cheddar cheese (3 1/2 oz.)	610
hot dog (1)	627
margarine (3 1/2 oz.)	800
butter, salted (3 1/2 oz.)	870
dill pickle (1 medium)	928
tomato ketchup (3 1/2 oz.)	1120
salt (one teaspoon)	2132

If you are eating a typical American diet, you are probably consuming the equivalent of about two to three teaspoons of sodium a day. As prevalent as sodium is, however, our taste for it is largely acquired. For that reason, if you become accustomed to eating foods with salt, it may take a bit of time to re-educate your sense of taste. However, many individuals who conscientiously limit their salt intake later report that they stop missing it.

Just how important is it to wean yourself from sodium? A growing number of studies show that just by cutting back on the amount of sodium you consume, you may be able to decrease your blood pressure.

Population studies have examined societies that consume low amounts of salt. Investigators have found that these people have a very low incidence of hypertension. The Eskimos in Alaska, the Tarahumara Indians of northern Mexico, and the Melanesian tribes of New Guinea consume low levels of sodium; not surprisingly, hypertension is extremely rare among them and does not become more prevalent as people age. By contrast, although many eating habits in Japan are excellent for cardiovascular health, in areas like northern Japan, where salt consumption is much higher than even in the United States, hypertension is quite commonplace.

Even so, some researchers remain unconvinced that there is a cause-and-effect relationship between sodium and blood pressure. In fact, there have been mixed findings in the medical literature. Many studies have found that a moderate reduction of dietary sodium resulted in a modest decline in blood pressure, averaging about 7 mm Hg in the systolic value; in other studies, patients have not experienced any significant change in blood pressure readings. One possible explanation for this may be that some individuals are genetically predisposed to be salt-sensitive, while others are not. We know from animal research that there are at least two distinct types of rats: some, the ALR and SHR strains, show significant increases in blood pressure with salt intake, while salt has no effect on the blood pressure of others.

According to Dr. James Nora, author of *The Whole Heart Book*, salt-sensitivity may be a complex interaction among hereditary factors, the kidneys, sodium, blood volume, blood chemistry, hormones, and stress. If you begin with unfavorable heredity, and subject the rat to stress and salt, it will develop hypertension. High blood pressure leads to stroke in the SHR strain, and to plaques in the blood vessels and often heart attacks in the ALR strain. Genetically, people may not be the same; that is, some may be more sensitive to the effects of salt than others.

Here are some other findings from recent studies:

> In one often-cited study, volunteers kept their daily intake of sodium at a modest level. This was enough to reduce their blood pressure values. Among patients with mild hyper-

tension—diastolic pressure between 90 and 114 mm Hg—85 percent experienced declines in diastolic pressure to less than 90 mm Hg.

The Australian National Health and Medical Research Council Dietary Salt Study involved 103 patients, about half of whom were placed on a low-salt diet. When the study began, this low-salt group had an average blood pressure of 155/95 mm Hg. On the low-salt program, these individuals experienced blood pressure declines of 5.5 to 2.8 mm Hg.

In a study conducted in Italy, 60 hypertensives were placed on a low-sodium/high-potassium diet. Their sodium intake was reduced about 38 percent and their potassium consumption was increased 63 percent, compared to a control diet. The results: The low-sodium high-potassium regimen resulted in significant declines in blood pressure, averaging 17 mm Hg in systolic values and 6 mm Hg in diastolic. These reductions occurred over a fourteen-day period.

The bottom line on sodium is that if you have high blood pressure, cutting back on sodium may not be the magic bullet that can single-handedly bring your problem under control. However, if you are salt-sensitive—a so-called "sodium reactor"—limiting salt can be an important part of your effort to normalize your blood pressure. If salt-sensitive individuals douse their vegetables with salt, night after night, their blood pressure will soar; their bodies do a poor job of excreting the excess sodium in their diet, and their blood pressure pays the price. On the other side of the coin, if these individuals cut back on their sodium consumption, their blood pressure will decline.

For individuals who are salt-sensitive, a major benefit of reducing sodium consumption is that they are frequently able to cut back on the amount of antihypertensive medication they take, **under their doctor's guidance.** One study showed that when sodium intake was significantly reduced, 80 percent of patients were able to either eliminate or significantly reduce the dosage of their medication.

As has already been suggested, however, there are also people for whom sodium seems to have little effect. Whether these people consume modest or large amounts of salt, their blood pressure does not respond one way or the other.

If you are salt-sensitive, take an assertive approach to the sodium issue. Many people with mild to moderate hypertension experience improvements in their blood pressure after even modest restrictions in their sodium intake, such as keeping their daily sodium intake at no more than two grams, or about one teaspoon of table salt.

How to Reduce Sodium Intake

How can you start reducing sodium in your diet? Here are some recommendations:

Choose fresh foods rather than packaged, canned or frozen items. Sodium is found in canned vegetables, gravies, salad dressings, and frozen entrees, although a growing number of food manufacturers are producing "low sodium" versions of their popular products. By contrast, not only do fresh foods have low amounts of sodium, they are also richer in protective vitamins and minerals.

Read food labels carefully. Salt is an ingredient in almost all processed foods. When you see the words salt or sodium early in the ingredients list, keep it out of your shopping cart (since ingredients are listed in descending order by weight).

Cut back on high-sodium foods such as ham, bacon, smoked or cured meats, canned soups, pickles, pretzels, and salted chips, nuts, and crackers. If you shop conscientiously, you can find low-salt frozen foods, soups and cereals, and unsalted nuts. For snacks, switch to healthy foods like **unsalted** air-popped popcorn, fruit, carrot sticks, or cauliflower wedges.

In the kitchen or at the dining-room table, use your salt shaker sparingly, if at all.

When seasoning food, replace salt with garlic, onions, herbs, and spices. Flavor or marinate your food with freshly-squeezed lemon or lime juice, apple cider vinegar, or aged gourmet balsamic vinegar.

When eating out, choose cooked-to-order foods over preprepared or fast food meals. Ask your server to "hold" the salt and sauces (MSG or soy sauce) and substitute garlic and herbs.

Moving toward a lower-salt diet can initially take some creative planning and substituting. If your food doesn't taste as good as you'd like, become more adventuresome in your use of herbs and spices. Your local chapter of the American Heart Association or health-conscious cookbooks can make the transition easier by supplying you with herb-oriented, low-salt recipes. With creative use of spices, you will soon begin to enjoy the natural taste of food and wonder why you relied so heavily on salt for so long.

THE BENEFITS OF DIETARY POTASSIUM

The average human body contains a healthy supply of potassium— about 9 ounces in a 150-pound man or woman. Your body needs potassium to survive, because it helps to maintain a balance between bodily fluids and cells. Potassium also assists nerves and muscles, including the heart, to function properly.

According to the 1988 report of the Joint National Committee on Detection, Evaluation, and Treatment of High Blood Pressure, there's another important role for potassium—namely, a high potassium intake (three to four grams a day) can help reduce your blood pressure. Although many people know that sodium can raise blood pressure in some individuals, there is less public awareness that potassium actually might be able to counteract some of that effect.

A study called the Health and Nutrition Examination Survey (HANES) has shown that potassium may help prevent high blood pressure. Individuals in the HANES study who consumed less than 1200 mg of potassium per day had twice the incidence of hypertension as those people with a potassium intake above 3600 mg.

A twelve-year-long study conducted by researchers in Rancho Bernardo, California, showed a 40 percent drop in stroke-related deaths among individuals consuming an extra 400 mg of potassium a day (a banana or a glass of skim milk). Women whose total potassium intake was less than 1900 mg per day had more than twice the chance of dying of a stroke than women who consumed more than 1900 mg.

For most of human history, our ancestors were on high-potassium, low-salt diets. However, in the last hundred years, this has changed, due to a 20-fold increase in sodium consumption, along with a potassium intake that is now about one-third of its previous level. Consequently, the 1 to 40 ratio of sodium-to-potassium of our early ancestors has been replaced by a 2 to 1 ratio!

How does potassium reduce blood pressure readings? At this point, the explanations are only speculative. Some researchers believe that high potassium levels can block the absorption of sodium by the kidneys. Others say that potassium may work like a diuretic, lowering the volume of blood plasma and thus decreasing blood pressure.

Whatever the mechanism, raising your potassium intake—while cutting back on your sodium consumption—makes good sense if your goal is lowering blood pressure and improving cardiovascular health. This means eating plenty of high-potassium foods, including certain fruits, leafy vegetables, and whole-grain products. If you buy and consume fresh bananas, oranges, apples, cantaloupe, nectarines, potatoes, peas, tomatoes, and legumes, you are on the right track. However, if you are considering taking potassium supplements, first consult your doctor. Certain patients—such as those with kidney problems, and people taking certain types of drugs, including potassium-sparing diuretics—may not be good candidates for this supplementation.

POTASSIUM CONTENT OF COMMON FOODS _____

	mg of potassium
brown rice (cooked, 1 cup)	278
haddock (3 oz.)	296
tomato (raw, 1 medium)	300
carrots (cooked, 1 cup)	344
milk (skim, 1 cup)	406
banana (1 medium)	440
chicken (1/2 broiler)	483
orange juice (1 cup)	496
sardines (3 oz., canned)	502
yogurt (plain, low-fat, 1 cup)	531
cantaloupe (1/2)	682
spinach (cooked, 1 cup)	688
dry beans (cooked, 1 cup)	749
potato (baked, medium)	782
apricots (dried, 1 cup)	1273
avocado (1)	1836

THE BENEFITS OF DIETARY CALCIUM

Calcium is the most prevalent mineral in the human body. It is essential for the formation and maintenance of healthy bones; more than 97 percent of the calcium in the body is present in the skeleton and teeth. When older individuals, women as well as men, experience the bone-thinning disease called *osteoporosis*, additional calcium in their diet, along with weight-bearing exercise, is often the best way to arrest the progression of this disorder. Of course, *preventing* osteoporosis would be even better, and is possible if you eat a diet rich in calcium and exercise regularly over your entire lifespan. Sufficient dietary calcium can keep this valuable mineral from being leached from the bones.

In recent years, researchers have also looked at the role that calcium might play in controlling blood pressure. There is some evidence pointing to a link between this mineral and hypertension. In studies of large populations in Honolulu and Puerto Rico, for example, the higher the calcium intake, the lower the average blood pressure.

A dietary review of 12,411 persons participating in the HANES study revealed that hypertensives had diets lower in calcium—as well as low levels of potassium, vitamin C and vitamin A—than people with normal blood pressure readings.

When Dr. David McCarron and other researchers at the Oregon Health Sciences University looked at calcium consumption in both hypertensives and normal individuals, the only significant difference between the two groups was that the hypertensives ingested an average of 25 percent less calcium than those with normal readings. In a separate study by the same investigators, when individuals with mild hypertension took one gram per day of oral calcium supplements for eight weeks, they experienced a lowering of both their systolic (5.6 mm Hg) and diastolic (2.3 mm Hg) blood pressures.

A four-year study by Dr. Nancy E. Johnson at the University of Wisconsin on the effects of calcium supplementation found a 13 mm Hg decline in systolic blood pressure among medication-taking hypertensives who also consumed calcium supplements. At the same time, a separate group of hypertensives on medication who did **not** take supplements experienced a 7 mm Hg **rise** in their systolic pressure. A third group of patients—those with **normal** blood pressure who took calcium supplements—experienced no change in their blood pressure.

There have been some intriguing animal studies as well, showing that high calcium diets may cause greater amounts of sodium to be secreted. This may be one of the mechanisms by which calcium can help reduce high blood pressure.

The results of tissue and cellular experiments are also worth noting. They have demonstrated that increased calcium may relax the smooth muscles in blood vessels. As calcium plays a role in the vasodilation of constricted blood vessels—that is, as it expands the vessels and allows a freer flow of blood—it decreases the pressure of the blood on arterial walls.

It may be too early to recommend that **all** hypertensives routinely take calcium supplements in hopes of controlling blood pressure. Nevertheless, it makes sense to at least meet the recommended daily allowance of calcium—800 to 1,200 mg a day. Women are advised to consume a minimum of 1,200 mg a day, and even more during pregnancy and while nursing.

Where should you get your calcium? In the supermarket, your choices seem almost endless. This mineral has been added to everything from orange juice to bread to breakfast cereals. However, there are better, more natural sources of calcium. Nonfat milk and other dairy products are particularly excellent foods in which to find calcium. Some nondairy foods, such as kale, collard greens, sardines, beans, spinach, and broccoli, also contain high amounts of calcium.

CALCIUM CONTENT OF COMMON FOODS ————————

	mg of calcium
corn muffin (1 medium)	45
orange (1 medium)	54
pinto beans (1 cup)	70
clams (1 cup)	110
okra (1 cup)	120
broccoli (1 cup, cooked)	136
kale (1 cup, cooked)	148
spinach (1 cup, cooked)	212
cheddar cheese (1 oz.)	213
oysters (1 cup)	227
swiss cheese (1 oz.)	262
collard greens (1 cup)	290
milk (skim, 1 cup)	296
sardines (3 oz., with bones)	372

Many doctors are now recommending calcium or multimineral tablets for their patients. If you do choose to use supplements, calcium carbonate, gluconate, or lactate are usually preferable to oyster-shell calcium, bone meal, and dolomite which (unless carefully tested) may contain trace amounts of lead. Calcium, in order to be assimilated, should be taken in conjunction with magnesium in about a 2 to 1 ratio—that is, twice as much calcium as magnesium. Multimineral supplements that supply calcium, magnesium, potassium, and other trace minerals that may be beneficial to your health are readily available.

No matter how you get your calcium, it is best not to overdo it. In a very small number of people, large amounts of calcium can put them at risk for developing kidney stones. If you have a problem with kidney stones, the stones can be analyzed to determine whether you are one of those people who needs to be careful about calcium consumption. Given the great health benefits of calcium, it is better not to needlessly deprive yourself of this important mineral.

THE BENEFITS OF DIETARY MAGNESIUM

Magnesium is a part of every cell in the body. It permits the nervous system to work efficiently by helping to transmit nerve impulses. It also ensures that various enzyme networks in the body function properly.

Magnesium, along with calcium, is considered one of the "anti-stress" minerals because of its calming effect. Magnesium may also play an important role in lowering blood pressure as well as protect the electrical stability of your heart. A number of studies indicate that even mild deficiencies in magnesium can contribute to high blood pressure, heart arrhythmias, and heart attacks. Yet most Americans consume only about 40 percent of the U.S. Recommended Daily Allowance (USRDA) for magnesium, which is presently 300 mg for women and 350 mg for men.

One of the largest magnesium research studies was conducted at Harvard Medical School and Brigham and Women's Hospital in Boston. Researchers evaluated diet and blood pressure in 58,218 women and concluded that magnesium was inversely associated with blood pressure—that is, as magnesium intake rose, blood pressure declined. Those women who received greater doses of magnesium developed less hypertension than women consuming smaller amounts in their diet.

Researchers with the Honolulu Heart study looked at the relationship of 61 nutritional factors—including magnesium—in 615 Hawaiian men, and their effect on high blood pressure. The researchers found that **more than any other nutrient,** increased magnesium levels were associated with a lowered incidence of hypertension.

A third study, headed by Dr. Thomas Dyckner, examined the effects of magnesium supplementation on 20 individuals with hypertension and/or congestive heart failure, and compared them with a control group who did not receive magnesium. After six months, the people who took magnesium showed a decline in systolic blood pressure from 152 mm Hg to 140 mm Hg, while the controls did not experience any change.

How does magnesium work? Experimental research indicates that magnesium may cause the arteries to relax, while a lack of this mineral can lead to their contraction. Thus, magnesium may help lower blood pressure by relaxing muscles in the blood vessel walls, thereby reducing the peripheral resistance that plays a role in hypertension. When Dr. William Mroczek and other scientists investigated the effects of intravenously-administered magnesium, they found a 35 percent decline in peripheral resistance in hypertensives, compared to only a 20 percent reduction in persons with normal blood pressure.

As I've already mentioned, if you supplement your diet with calcium, make sure you are also consuming adequate magnesium. These two minerals work synergistically, so it is best to try to keep your calcium and magnesium intake at about a 2 to 1 ratio. With high levels of calcium (above 1300 mg per day), your body may experience magnesium depletion unless you are also taking additional magnesium.

Here are some other facts about magnesium to keep in mind:

If your diet is high in phosphates—found in protein and soft drinks—this may interfere with the absorption of magnesium. You might need to increase your intake of magnesium.

Magnesium may help buffer your heart against the stress hormone, adrenaline. According to animal studies, during times of stress, adrenaline is released in the body, which can cause damage to the arteries. However, when laboratory animals were given magnesium supplements, they were protected from the injuries that adrenaline can cause.

As was pointed out earlier, magnesium can play a significant role in stabilizing the electrical activity of the heart. When there are low levels of magnesium, the heart is more vulnerable to arrhythmias. While about 1 in 20 healthy people have some irregularity in their heart rhythm—such as a periodic skipped beat—an arrhythmia in an individual recovering from a heart attack can be potentially life-threatening. Preliminary research indicates that magnesium can calm these arrhythmias. In fact, researchers found many years ago that infusions of magnesium during open heart surgery can minimize the chances of fibrillation (a disorganization of the heart's electrical activity that keeps it from contracting properly and can cause sudden death).

By stabilizing abnormalities in the heart's rhythm, magnesium can normalize irregular electrocardiograms. When researchers gave 240 to 360 mg of a form of magnesium to 25 patients over a two-year period, the QT and QU intervals (measurable patterns) on their ECGs—which can be associated with sudden death when they are abnormal—showed a return to a healthy pattern.

The results of a Danish study involving 130 heart attack patients delivered a strong endorsement for magnesium. When the study started, all of these patients had low-to-average magnesium levels. One group was given supplements of magnesium, while another received sugar water. About one-half of those taking the placebo experienced arrhythmias, and 7 of 74 of these patients died. In contrast, only about one-quarter of the magnesium group had arrhythmias, resulting in 2 deaths among 56 patients.

Some studies indicate that magnesium helps prevent enlargement of the heart and the death of heart tissue.

If your diet is low in magnesium, this can lead to a potassium deficiency as well. On the other hand, regular consumption of magnesium supplements can increase the amount of potassium in the cells of the body.

If you are taking diuretics, you may have a magnesium—as well as potassium—depletion as a side effect of this drug. One study showed that when individuals on long-term diuretic therapy were given 365 mg of magnesium a day, their systolic and diastolic blood pressure readings decreased an average of 12 and 8 mm Hg, respectively, over a six-month period.

Even so, not all diuretics cause this problem. Yes, chlorothiazide (Diuril) and other thiazide-based diuretics—as well as the stronger diuretic called furosemide (Lasix)—do deplete the body's supply of magnesium. But others, including spironolactone (Aldalctone), have no such negative impact. Please check with your doctor as to whether supplemental magnesium (as well as potassium and calcium) are advisable in conjunction with the particular antihypertensive medication you are taking.

Despite the important roles it plays, magnesium has received less attention than calcium in particular. One problem is the difficulty in using blood tests to determine the adequacy of an individual's magnesium level. Paradoxically, just when tissue concentrations of magnesium are at their lowest, blood levels of magnesium are elevated. In one study, researchers evaluated the levels of magnesium in the blood and in the tissue in 25 patients on diuretics. They found that in 15 of these subjects, even though there was a deficiency of magnesium in the tissues, the blood magnesium content was normal.

If you are concerned about blood pressure and your heart, make magnesium-rich foods a regular part of your diet. The following chart shows where you can find magnesium.

MAGNESIUM CONTENT OF COMMON FOODS ―――――――――

	mg of magnesium
kelp (1 tablespoon)	104
almonds (1/4 cup)	96
wheat germ (1/4 cup)	91
oatmeal (1 cup, cooked)	56
brown rice (1/4 cup, raw)	43
collard greens (1/2 cup)	42
avocado (1/2)	39
whole wheat flour (1/4 cup)	34
banana (1)	33
yams (1/2 cup)	31

	mg of magnesium
cantaloupe (1/2)	28
green peas (1/2 cup)	25
ricotta cheese, part skim (1/2 cup)	18
dates (5)	15
liver (3 oz.)	11

THE BENEFITS OF DIETARY CHROMIUM

If you have atherosclerosis, diabetes, or hyperglycemia (glucose intolerance), you may also have a chromium deficiency. Chromium is an essential part of the Glucose Tolerance Factor (GTF)—an indicator of your capacity to assimilate sugars—which is needed for proper insulin function and glucose metabolism.

An article published in the journal *Pysiological Review* reported that a deficiency in chromium can cause changes in the body similar to adult-onset diabetes, including poor glucose tolerance, an elevated cholesterol count, and a rise in the fasting glucose levels (the measurement of a person's blood glucose level after a pure glucose solution is ingested following an all-night fast). Supplementing the diet with chromium, however, can reverse these negative effects. When chromium is added to the diet, both blood cholesterol levels and the rate of atherosclerosis decrease. Researchers at Mercy Hospital and Medical Center in San Diego discovered that chromium supplements (200 micrograms a day) could raise HDL cholesterol and reduce LDL cholesterol in a little more than a month.

Even so, surveys show that chromium consumption in the United States is low compared to nations where diabetes and atherosclerosis are less common. Chromium is needed only in micro amounts—you can find 200 micrograms of inorganic chromium in about 10 to 20 grams of brewers yeast or about 2 to 3 tablespoons a day. Chromium is also present in foods like vegetables, whole grains, legumes, and fresh fruit.

WHAT ABOUT VITAMIN SUPPLEMENTS?

For years, vitamin pills have been immersed in controversy. Some people swear that vitamins are essential for maintaining good health or that they are all that stands between themselves and serious illness. Others insist that if you eat well-balanced meals, you're only wasting your money by buying and using vitamin supplements.

What's the truth? It probably lies somewhere in-between. Vitamins are required by the body for the formation of nervous-system chemicals, blood cells, hormones, and many other compounds. However, the body does not manufacture vitamins, except for vitamin D, and you therefore need to get them from your diet.

Ideally, you should be able to get all the vitamins you require from the foods you eat. However, foods are not what they used to be. Too many of them are processed, refined, and sprayed with chemicals. When that happens, vitamins are often destroyed, and thus, deficiencies are not uncommon.

To further complicate matters, the United States Recommended Daily Allowance (RDA) of vitamins is somewhat suspect. These RDAs are **not** the vitamin intake necessary to promote optimal health; instead, they are the levels required to prevent nutritional deficiencies. So while the RDAs may be a good starting point, they should not be your "vitamin bible," if your goal is to keep yourself in the best possible health.

Many people think of vitamin and mineral supplements as a type of "insurance policy." You may not need them on a given day or week, but during those times when you neglect your diet a little, when you're under a lot of stress, or when you're recovering from an illness, they may provide the backup nutrients you need to maintain good health.

Even so, it is better not to get carried away with vitamins, particularly the fat-soluble ones—vitamins A, D, E, and K—which can be dangerous if taken in excessive doses. Nevertheless, the case **for** vitamins is becoming stronger. A growing number of studies shows that vitamins are critical to good health, and may even play a role in normalizing blood pressure and preventing heart disease. As with minerals, the evidence is not yet conclusive, but it has become persuasive enough that you should be aware of the possibilities as you fine-tune your personal program to normalize your blood pressure.

VITAMIN C

Vitamin C has been championed for its role in the prevention and treatment of many illnesses—ranging from cancer to the common cold—as well as in helping wounds to heal, in forming brain chemicals, and synthesizing proteins. Vitamin C can help keep teeth and bones strong and contribute to the flexibility and well-being of vein and capillary walls.

Researchers, however, know much less about vitamin C's ability to help prevent coronary heart disease. Even so, there is a growing body of research indicating that vitamin C may have a place in cardiovascular care.

A 20-country study found a rise in heart disease deaths as the intake of fruits and vegetables—the main source of vitamin C—declined. A separate 30-nation study showed similar results: The incidence of heart disease decreased as the consumption of vitamin-rich vegetables and grains went up.

As discussed earlier, the importance of low cholesterol to a healthy heart is well-established. Many studies have concluded that blood cholesterol levels decline in response to seasonal increases in vitamin C intake. Other research indicates that when vitamin C consumption is low, blood cholesterol rises.

Emil Ginter, an authority on vitamin C and coronary vascular disease, reviewed thirteen clinical trials that evaluated the relationship between vitamin C and cholesterol. In his article in the prestigious British journal *Lancet,* Dr. Ginter observed that cholesterol levels above 200 mg/dl decreased when vitamin C was added to the diet; by contrast, in people with cholesterol readings below 200 mg/dl, cholesterol levels did not change with the addition of vitamin C. Seven separate controlled studies have concurred that vitamin C supplementation, in amounts above 500 mg per day, produced decreases in cholesterol for individuals whose cholesterol levels were initially greater than 200 mg/dl.

While vitamin C supplements are widely available in supermarkets and pharmacies, the richest dietary sources are citrus fruits, green and red peppers, berries, melons, tomatoes, tropical fruits, green leafy vegetables, broccoli, cauliflower, and potatoes. On average, one cup of each of these foods provides about 100 mg of vitamin C.

Even though the minimum RDA for vitamin C is 60 mg, many nutritional surveys indicate that 30 to 50 percent of the U.S. population consume less than 45 mg daily. Some researchers have advised changing the RDA to 200 mg or 300 mg for optimal health. A number of nutritionists now recommend even more—1000 mg (1 gram) or more, depending on the specific individual's health status. Fortunately, vitamin C is water-soluble. If you take more than your body needs or can utilize, you merely eliminate it.

Two caveats: Some research suggests that high doses of vitamin C (more than 2 grams a day) should be taken in conjunction with at least 2 mg of dietary copper, since animal studies and one human trial suggest that high-dose vitamin C can deplete copper levels in the body. Zinc supplements can also deplete copper and require some micro-supplementation of copper (2 mg per day).

Also, a very small number of people might develop kidney stones with long-term, high-dose vitamin C consumption. Nevertheless, one study found that even megadoses (ten grams a day) of vitamin C created only mild increases in the body's excretion of the substance that can lead to kidney stones. Again, stone analysis will help you and your physician determine if limiting vitamin C would be advisable for you. But for most individuals, the benefits of vitamin C outweigh the risks.

VITAMIN E AND SELENIUM

Vitamin E and selenium are both *antioxidants:* they prevent oxidation, which can not only turn foods rancid, but also permits benign chemicals in the body to become dangerous ones. The presence of vitamin E and selenium also interferes with the oxidation of polyunsaturated fats and, in the process, prevents damage to the cell membranes. As your fat— particularly polyunsaturated fat—intake rises, so should your consumption of vitamin E.

Vitamin E may be especially beneficial to people with angina pain. Because this vitamin enables us to utilize oxygen more efficiently, it can actually help reduce angina, which is literally oxygen-deprived heart cells crying out for air.

Clinical trials have shown that vitamin E also has potential benefits for HDL cholesterol levels. In a small study by Dr. William Hermann, 10 patients at Memorial City General Hospital in Houston received 600 IU of vitamin E per day. HDL values soared an average of 375 percent after 40 days in patients with initially low levels; while HDL increased 168 percent in patients who started with normal levels. Although the results of most subsequent studies have not been as impressive, some research does confirm that vitamin E may raise HDL levels, particularly in younger patients with low HDL values. Rich sources of vitamin E include whole grain breads and cereals, leafy green vegetables, dried beans, vegetable oils, wheat germ, and nuts.

A deficiency of selenium has also been linked to cardiovascular disease. In parts of the United States where selenium is present in high amounts, there is a lower incidence of deaths from coronary vascular disease. In Finland, researchers discovered that people who suffered heart attacks tended to have lower selenium levels in their blood than people who did not have heart attacks; individuals with lower blood selenium levels (under 34 μg/ml) had nearly 7 times the risk of death from heart disease as people with higher selenium levels (over 45 μg/ml).

Keep in mind, however, that researchers generally recommend that you do not exceed 200 μg per day of selenium, since studies are still being conducted on the effects of high intakes of this mineral. The best food sources of selenium are seafood, chicken, onions, garlic, milk, whole grain cereals, and meat.

NIACIN AND THE OTHER B VITAMINS

Over the last 35 years, studies have shown that niacin or nicotinic acid (vitamin B_3)—in doses above 1000 mg—can help reduce cholesterol and triglyceride levels.

A study involving 160 individuals with high blood cholesterol levels discovered that nicotinic acid reduced cholesterol levels an average of 26 percent.

In the Coronary Drug project, 1100 people with coronary heart disease took 3000 mg of nicotinic acid a day; they experienced a 10 percent reduction in their cholesterol values and a 26 percent decline in their triglyceride levels, compared to a group taking placebo.

Dr. David Blankenhorn headed up a two-year study at the University of Southern California, examining niacin in combination with colestipol, a cholesterol-lowering drug. The research showed that LDL ("bad") cholesterol levels plummeted 43 percent on these substances, while HDL ("good") cholesterol levels increased 37 percent. Even more impressive, atherosclerotic plaques regressed in 16 percent of the individuals, while the disease process in most of the other patients slowed.

While time-release capsules were previously thought to be a good choice because they prevent the uncomfortable niacin flush that often accompanies niacin consumption, recent research indicates that time-release may not be the best choice after all, because it can also contribute to liver damage.

Before you begin taking niacin, it is absolutely essential that you first check with your doctor. Used in the large amounts necessary to achieve improvements in cholesterol levels, niacin becomes a drug and thus requires regular medical monitoring, including liver function tests and glucose and uric acid tests every three to six months. In general, niacin therapy should be avoided by individuals with liver damage— either from hepatitis, heavy drinking, or other problems, because of the excessive strain it places on the liver. People with diabetes, severe heart arrhythmias, peptic ulcers, and gout are generally not considered candidates for niacin therapy.

Several other B vitamins are worthy of mention, too. Some research indicates that pyridoxine (vitamin B_6) may interfere with the grouping together of platelets (sticky blood cells that assist in clotting), thus preventing clotting that is associated with heart attacks and strokes. Animal studies show that a diet deficient in vitamin B_6 is associated with atherosclerosis.

Vitamin B₁ (thiamine) plays a role in the proper functioning of the nervous and digestive systems. Vitamin B₂ (riboflavin) helps the body make the best use of oxygen, while also promoting healthy skin and eyes.

In fact, the entire complex of B vitamins are utilized in nearly every cell of the body. Some research indicates that the body's need for B vitamins rises during stressful periods—and that the vitamins work best in tandem with one another. If even one of them is deficient, the others may function at sub-optimal levels. In orthomolecular medicine, which specializes in the nutritional treatment of disease, high dosages of B vitamins have been helpful in treating nervous tension, irritability, anxiety, and depression.

Foods like chicken, split peas, avocado, brewer's yeast, prunes, sweet potatoes, and broccoli are good sources of the B vitamins. If you are eating a diet rich in complex carbohydrates along with some animal protein, you will probably be getting all the vitamin B you need, although supplementation of a balanced B complex—which contains all of the B vitamins—may be advisable during times of stress.

VITAMIN D

Is vitamin D actually a "vitamin?" Not really. More accurately, it could be labeled a steroid hormone, and its effect on the body could be hazardous to your long-term cardiovascular health if your combined intake each day is greater that 400 mg. In excessive amounts, vitamin D can contribute to the development of atherosclerosis. Animal studies show that vitamin D is associated with atherosclerosis of the left descending coronary artery—the most ominous site of arterial blockage; so serious, in fact, that blockage in this area can make an individual a candidate for coronary bypass surgery.

Only a few foods—such as butter, eggs, and fish liver oils—contain vitamin D. However, when your skin is exposed to the sun, your body synthesizes vitamin D from cholesterol; that is usually all the vitamin D you need. As a general rule, if you receive adequate sun exposure—even just 10 to 15 minutes, two to three times a week—on the face, hands and arms—there is really no need for supplemental vitamin D. However, to prevent premature aging of the skin and skin cancer, it is advisable to stay out of the sun between 11:00 A.M. and 3:00 P.M. and use a sunscreen with a Sun Protection Factor (SPF) of at least 15 if you plan to be out in the sun for a prolonged period of time.

Initially, vitamin D was added to food products to prevent rickets. But only 100 mg a day is sufficient to prevent this disease and most people consume more than that, thanks to the vitamin's routine addition to milk, cereals, processed foods, and many other supermarket items. In fact, most of us actually consume **too much** vitamin D. Although the RDA for this vitamin is 400 IU, many adults and children take in twice that amount or more. Thus, it may be wise to limit your vitamin D intake.

CONCLUSIONS

As much as possible, obtain your vitamins and minerals from the foods in your diet. Supplements are not a substitute for cardiowise nutritional habits; however, because you may not always be getting the best nutrition—or since your nutritional needs may increase if you are under stress—supplements are useful for many people and are freer of side effects than high blood pressure medications. Even so, continue to rely primarily on vitamin- and mineral-rich foods; if you select them wisely, they can contribute significantly to lowering your blood pressure and guarding your cardiovascular health.

CHAPTER 14

Tipping the Scales in Your Favor: What If You Need to Lose Weight?

We have evidence that weight loss, sodium restriction, and relief of stress will lower the blood pressure of those already hypertensive.

—NORMAN KAPLAN, M.D.
University of Texas
Southwestern Medical
Center

THE LAST TIME YOU VISITED YOUR DOCTOR, did he or she suggest that you "need to lose a few pounds?" If you are carrying some excess weight, and you also have hypertension, your doctor's advice makes sense. Hypertension is about twice as common among obese individuals as it is among people of normal weight. Obesity places extra strain on your heart and cardiovascular system, forcing them to work harder and contributing to your high blood pressure. Each extra pound of fatty tissue requires an additional mile of capillaries to nourish it.

The average American gains about 1 to 2 pounds a year between the ages of 20 and 50, coinciding with a gradual slowing of their metabolic rate of about 7 percent per decade. While your bathroom scale can tell you what you weigh, it can't determine what percentage of your body weight is fat as opposed to lean muscle mass, which does not create the risk of coronary heart disease. You will need either an underwater weighing or a skin-fold measurement, available at many hospitals and health clubs, for an accurate determination of how much body fat you are carrying.

Your lean muscle mass actually burns calories and determines how much you can eat. If two people eat the same number of calories, the one with the **least** lean body mass will tend to gain the most weight. By eating right, you can maintain or increase your lean muscle mass while decreasing excess fat.

To further complicate the picture, researchers involved in the Honolulu Heart study discovered that **where** you carry your body fat makes a difference in your cardiovascular risk—that is, if your excess pounds have accumulated primarily on the front of the abdomen, you have twice the chance of having a heart attack as people whose fat is concentrated on the hips, thighs, or sides of the torso. The good news is that by shedding a few excess pounds, you can help get your blood pressure under control. The Framingham Heart study found that when individuals lost 10 percent of their body weight—15 pounds in a 150-pound woman, for example—systolic blood pressure declined an average of 5 mm Hg. In the Chicago Coronary Prevention Evaluation program, overweight men with mild hypertension lost an average of 12 pounds—a modest weight reduction, but one that produced a decline in both systolic and diastolic pressure to **normal** levels.

In another study, investigators in Israel put 81 obese, hypertensive volunteers on low-calorie diets that ranged from 800 to 1200 calories per day. After 2 months, these individuals had lost an average of more than 20 pounds. At the same time, their systolic blood pressure declined 26 mm Hg, while their diastolic readings fell 20 mm Hg. These declines were attributed solely to weight loss, since sodium intake was not reduced in the study population.

If you have hypertension and are even slightly overweight, your blood pressure will probably benefit from shedding that excess fat. When that happens your doctor may be able to reduce your dosage of antihypertensive medication, or even eliminate drugs completely.

SOUND STRATEGIES FOR SHEDDING FAT

If you have tried losing weight in the past, you know that it is a challenge—and keeping the pounds off can be even more difficult. At first glance, the formula for weight loss seems like a simple one: Burn up more calories than you take in through your diet. However, it may require dedication to some proven strategies for you to win the losing battle. To bring your weight under control and keep it there, here are some sound strategies:

Rather than thinking in terms of a diet, plan and make some fundamental changes in your food selections and eating behavior. You probably will not be well served in the long run by a "crash" program; but you will benefit over a lifetime if you adopt commonsense, moderate nutritional habits that will assist you in normalizing and maintaining your preferred weight.

Avoid high-protein, low-carbohydrate diets that were once so fad-
dish. If you lose 10 pounds on one of these high-protein programs, three of those pounds will be water, which will quickly
return once you go off the diet. Even worse, these diets cause
muscle loss and less efficient calorie burning. For every pound of
fat you lose on a high-protein, low-carbohydrate diet, you might
lose nearly a pound of lean muscle mass.

Eat three meals a day, and incorporate a variety of foods into them,
using the basic guidelines you'll find in the nutrition chapters of
this book. Plan your meals so that most of your calories come
from complex carbohydrates—such as vegetables, fruits, and
grains—which are rich sources of fiber, vitamins, and minerals,
but have a lower caloric content than high-fat foods. Interestingly, if you get most of your calories from high complex-
carbohydrate foods rather than high-fat foods, fewer of those
calories will "go to fat." According to a 1984 study, when animals
were placed on a high-fat diet with 42 to 60 percent of their
calories coming from fat, they ended up obese, with 51 percent
body fat; by contrast, a control group consuming the same number of calories as part of a **low-fat** diet ended up with only 30
percent body fat. Fat calories may, in fact, be more fattening
than other kinds of calories.

Therefore, if weight management is your goal, it makes even more
sense to include fresh vegetables, fruits, and whole grains as part
of each meal. Choose fish, turkey, and chicken skinned before
cooking as your primary sources of animal protein, and keep
portion sizes moderate (three–four ounces). Eat red meat infre-
quently. For snacks, select air-popped popcorn, a cluster of ripe
grapes, or other fruit.

When you are hungry between means, fresh, raw, or steamed high-
fiber, low-calorie vegetables are an excellent choice. Take some
cut-up, raw vegetables with you for a low-calorie snack during
the day, and keep some eye-appealing, cut-up vegetables in the
refrigerator. For dressings, use herbs, lemons, vinegar and onions, or low-fat yogurt dip. Feeling comfortably full on vegetables will provide you with added ballast to diminish the
temptation to eat high-calorie, high-fat foods.

Rely on skim milk and nonfat dairy products instead of whole milk
and whole-milk products. Rather than butter, use a tablespoon
of monounsaturated oils for cooking. Bear in mind, however,
that oils in general should be used sparingly since they average
120 calories per teaspoon.

Minimize or eliminate empty calories from sugar, avoiding them
not only in the sugar bowl but in baked goods, desserts, soft

drinks, jams, sweetened juices, breakfast cereals, and other processed foods. Choose low-calorie, low-fat fruit, or fructose-
sweetened alternatives, and cut back on portion sizes. Think
substitution, **not** deprivation.

Eat your larger meals earlier in the day, and eat lighter later. At the
Aerobics Center in Dallas, overweight women on a 1200-calorie-
a-day diet consumed 25 percent of their calories at breakfast, 50
percent at lunch, and 25 percent at dinner; on this regimen, they
lost an average of 1 to 3 pounds per week.

Go grocery shopping on a full stomach so you won't be as tempted
to impulsively put unhealthy items into your cart. Shop around
the outer parts of the store first, where you'll tend to find the
fresh foods. Minimize temptations whenever possible; if a particular food isn't on your eating plan, don't buy it in the first
place. Keep it out of your shopping cart, your refrigerator, and
your cupboard—and off your plate.

Make tradeoffs. When you do eat a high-calorie, high-fat food,
counterbalance it by eating lower-calorie foods for the next few
meals and increasing your physical activity.

Keep an accurate diary of your eating habits for one week. Write
down the types and amounts of food you consume, the time of
day you eat, and how you feel before and after eating. When you
go back and review this diary, it will help you identify the high-
caloric food choices in your diet and substitute healthier, lower-
caloric alternatives. With a diary, many people find out for the
first time just how much they eat—including their constant nib-
bling while on the run, watching TV, or cooking. In the weeks
ahead, start assessing the calories on your plate **before** eating
them.

Make exercise a regular part of your life. Find a physical activity
you enjoy, and set aside time for it at least four to six times a
week. Exercise increases the synthesis of hundreds of enzymes
that help burn up calories and it raises your metabolic rate so you
become a better "fat burner," actually using up more calories
even when you're at rest because of your accelerated metabolism.
Regular exercise will also suppress your appetite.

If you diet **without** exercising, about 25 percent of the pounds lost
will be lean muscle mass—not fat—which is far from ideal. The
timing of your exercise can also help burn fat. If you exercise
regularly and schedule your workout no more than two hours
prior to the evening meal, you will lose more body fat than if you
exercise at other times of the day, apparently because you will
have raised your metabolic rate. Without exercise, your metabolism tends to slow down toward the end of the day. If you miss

your pre-dinner exercise, taking a half-hour walk after dinner can not only help keep your metabolism higher in the evening, but it can burn up an additional 200 calories, which could add up to a loss of about 20 pounds of excess fat in a year.

How vigorously should you exercise? To burn fat, plan moderate workouts—that is, activity at less than 80 percent of your target heart rate. If you exceed that 80 percent level, you will tend to burn pure glucose, not fat. (Chapter 16 provides both information and inspiration to help you accurately calculate your target heart rate zone and develop your own exercise program.)

Manage your stress. Stress not only tends to promote overeating and binge eating (often on high-fat or sugar-laden foods), it also releases hormones like adrenaline that stimulate insulin release and interfere with the breakdown of fat.

To help you lose excess fat and keep it off, adopt behavioral modification techniques. For instance, eat only when you're hungry, not just because it's "time for lunch." Take the edge off your hunger before sitting down to meals by first drinking a glass of water, low-salt tomato juice, or seltzer with a slice of lemon or lime. Place only as much food on your plate as you want to eat. Start with a big salad or raw or steamed vegetables before higher-calorie foods.

Eat slowly, setting your fork down occasionally between bites. If you eat with others, you will tend to eat more slowly because you will be talking between bites. Remember that it takes about 20 minutes for your body to register the sensation of being full and satisfied. When you're no longer hungry, stop eating and push the plate away.

Create and write down a series of both short-term and long-term weight goals, and chart your progress over time. A one- to two-pound loss per week is a sensible target. This gradual, steady approach to normalizing your weight will allow you to cultivate the new lifestyle habits that can help you maintain a lower, healthier weight. Remember, a rapid weight loss tends to be followed by weight gain ("the yo-yo syndrome"), which can ultimately decrease your lean muscle mass, making it easier for you to regain weight, again and again, and harder to lose it in the future.

Once a week, weigh yourself in the morning, before breakfast. Then review your progress and recommit yourself to your weight-loss objectives. Also, be sure to reward yourself as you attain your short- as well as longer-term goals—perhaps by buying yourself new clothes, a pair of walking, running, or aerobic shoes, a health magazine, or a new exercise videotape for the leaner, lighter you.

CHANGING YOUR SET POINT

The approach described in this chapter will help you change your *set point*, a concept borrowed from systems control theory (the way in which bodily systems regulate themselves) and based on the body's tendency to maintain its body fat at a certain level, even as its caloric consumption decreases. As you reduce your intake of calories, it may be difficult to lose fat, since the body instinctively slows down its fat-burning metabolism in order to maintain weight at a particular set point. This theory may explain in part why some very overweight individuals can eat relatively little and still gain weight, while their thinner friends can eat large amounts of food and remain lean.

This phenomenon is less than fair. Fortunately, however, you can recalibrate your set point to accept a lower amount of body fat as "normal" by eating foods high in complex carbohydrates, while limiting simple carbohydrates, sugars, and salt-laden foods; restricting the total calories you eat each day; exercising four to six times a week; and becoming more active in your daily life. Coincidentally, these same strategies will help you normalize your blood pressure.

THE FOOD-MOOD INTERACTION

Is much of what you eat related to mood management? A lot of eating—including what, when, and how much we consume—can be motivated by our need to manage our mood rather than by actual hunger.

We may reach for food to calm ourselves when we are concerned or anxious, or to lift our spirits when we are down or depressed.

In *Who Gets Sick: Thinking and Health*, Dr. Blair Justice says that since eating can provide short-term relief from psychological pain, our moods can influence what we eat. Studies, in fact, show that our emotional state, and our level of self-confidence or insecurity, plays a role in the types of food we choose. When individuals are depressed, anxious, or under constant stress, they frequently turn to "junk food;" people in greater control are more likely to rely on well-balanced meals.

Dr. Justice believes that when we chronically feel "down," we may decide to eat high-carbohydrate snacks, which can elevate levels of a brain chemical called serotonin and lift our mood. While snack foods can cause the release of more serotonin, large amounts of sweets appear to release another substance, endorphins, which can ease pain. Both serotonin and endorphin are natural ways to reduce sensitivity to pain.

Up to this point, using food to manage your moods may be the best way you have found to stave off whatever may feel distressing. However, a significant component of effective weight management is learning to cultivate methods for managing stress, discomfort, or anxiety in ways that maintain and build health, rather than perpetuating habits that can help you cope in the short-term but may harm you over time.

It is important to understand that less than desirable habits, fueled by your need to manage your mood rather than by hunger, can be changed more easily if you can identify your actual needs—which are important—and meet them in a way that will return your sense of control right where it belongs—within you.

Here is a five-step process that can help:

1. Identify and write down what is happening, how you feel, and what you are thinking or saying to yourself at those times you are tempted to eat too much or reach for high-fat, sugar- or salt-laden foods.
2. Generate a list of specific, self-care actions you can implement at these times, to replace your old, less desirable behavior. These alternatives should be at least as good as, if not better than, your former habits, and could include reaching for vegetables and fruits you have prepared, using your stress management skills, taking a walk or extra exercise class, or calling a friend.
3. Mentally rehearse your new self-care and eating behaviors when you wake up each morning. For some help with this technique, read the "Slimming Through Imaging" section that follows this five-step process.
4. Take advantage of every opportunity throughout the day to implement new, preferred behavior.
5. Take it one day at a time, and acknowledge each success you have.

SLIMMING THROUGH IMAGING

There is an additional strategy you can use to help normalize and maintain your preferred weight, which incorporates the relaxation and imaging exercises you learned earlier in the book.

Here's how it works: When you wake up each day, devote a few minutes to imagining yourself engaging in specific activities that will assist you in shedding extra pounds and maintaining a normal weight. Develop a multisensory imaging sequence—seeing, feeling, and hearing the "lighter, leaner, healthier you" engaging in healthy, cardiowise eating, exercise, and lifestyle habits.

As part of your imaging process, picture yourself making specific choices that will promote effective weight management. For example, visualize yourself grocery shopping. What are you putting into the cart?

When you open the refrigerator at home, what are you taking out? How are you preparing your food (are you cooking with salt and butter, or with a measured amount of olive oil)? What are you putting on your plate and on the table?

Imagine yourself eating in a restaurant: What types of food are you choosing? What healthy substitutions can you see yourself making? When you socialize with friends, are you making cardiowise food and beverage selections?

When you are upset or stressed, can you see, feel, and hear yourself actively choosing alternative ways of managing stress, such as taking time to breathe and relax, go for a walk, or call a friend? Can you picture yourself engaging in and enjoying regular exercise?

Can you imagine how much better you would feel carrying fewer pounds as you move? Are you exercising four to six times a week and enjoying it? Can you envision yourself admiring your leaner body, enjoying how well your clothes look on you—and how much better you look without clothes!

To help you successfully stay on course toward your goals, incorporate the following affirmation into your imagery process, which many HART patients have found helpful: "My body normalizes itself at its ideal weight of ____ pounds and adjusts its needs, habits and functions accordingly."

You may find that using this imagery and affirmation technique every day will contribute significantly to your slimming program.

Along the way, if you need support to stay on course, get it! There are many qualified, experienced therapists and nutritionists out there who can support you in achieving your goals. A variety of nation-wide programs are available, ranging from Weight Watchers to TOPS (Take Off Pounds Sensibly), that encourage a balanced diet and regular exercise.

Finally, once you reach your "ideal" weight, continue committing yourself to a fit, healthy lifestyle, accessible through good nutrition and regular exercise. This will help keep your weight—and, in turn, your blood pressure—right where you want it.

CHAPTER 15

A Brief Word About Smoking

*To cease smoking is the easiest thing I ever did. I ought to
know because I've done it a hundred times!*

—MARK TWAIN

MORE THAN 50 MILLION Americans smoke, despite the hazardous effects
of cigarettes upon health. When smokers enter the HART Program
and are asked why they continue to use cigarettes, they respond with a
variety of answers. For instance:

1. "I find it relaxing."
2. "It's an enjoyable habit. I've been doing it for years."
3. "It keeps me from overeating. If there's a cigarette in my mouth,
   I won't put food in it."
4. "I'm addicted. I want to stop, but I don't think I can."

At least in a general sense, most people know that smoking is unhealthy. Yet many never realistically confront the devastation that cigarettes can cause in their own lives—and how important it is to quit. In
1990, Surgeon General Antonia C. Novello put it succinctly: "Smoking
cessation represents the single most important step that smokers can
take to enhance the length and quality of their lives."

Let's look at the facts.

THE HEALTH CONSEQUENCES

What's the most common disease associated with smoking? Most people
answer lung cancer. A few might mention cancers of the mouth, throat,
esophagus, oral cavity, bladder, and pancreas. However, even though
the link between cigarettes and cancer is well-substantiated, smoking's
toll upon the cardiovascular system is even more ominous. Here's what
the American Heart Association says: "The bottom line is that about

350,000 deaths every year are attributed to smoking. And most of these deaths result, not from cancer, but from heart attack."

If you have high blood pressure, it is particularly important that you quit smoking. Although cigarettes don't cause hypertension, both smoking and high blood pressure are cardiovascular "risk factors" that, when combined, dramatically increase your chances of suffering a heart attack. If you also have high cholesterol, lead a sedentary lifestyle, have had a heart attack or stroke, eat a high-fat diet, take birth-control pills, have a family history of heart disease, or have diabetes, you are in even more danger.

The harmful gases and other byproducts of cigarettes show little mercy upon your lungs and cardiovascular system. Smoking actually causes short-term rises in both systolic and diastolic blood pressure. It also constricts the blood vessels, speeds up the heart rate, increases the stickiness of blood platelets and the risk of blood clotting, and interferes with the oxygen supply to the brain.

In coronary heart disease, the heart does not receive enough oxygen, and smoking only exacerbates that problem. Oxygen in the blood is carried by molecules of hemoglobin, a critical component of red blood cells. Among smokers, however, the carbon monoxide from cigarettes attaches so tightly to the hemoglobin that the transport of oxygen is hindered. As a result, smokers are at a higher risk for all serious cardiovascular problems, including strokes and heart attacks, which lead to premature disability and death.

YOU CAN QUIT

Confronted with evidence like this, in tandem with the toll most people feel smoking takes on their well-being, many people **do** stop smoking. In fact, **over 38 million adult Americans have quit.** If you have high blood pressure and you care about your health and well-being, why not make a commitment to join them? I am convinced that persons who smoke have their own inner sense of when it is time to quit. No one can force another person to stop, but being informed can help you set the time to stop that works for you.

Some people erroneously think that even if they successfully stop smoking, the benefits will be questionable. As one HART participant said, "I've been smoking for almost 30 years. I've probably already done so much damage to my heart and lungs that quitting now is not going to do me much good." However, **this is not the case.** Just days after your lungs have inhaled your last cigarette, your body starts to heal itself. Without doubt, **individuals who stop smoking live longer.** It's that simple.

Here are some of the statistics from the 1990 Surgeon General's report, *The Health Benefits of Smoking Cessation:*

> Just one year after quitting, your risk of smoking-related heart disease is reduced by one-half. After fifteen years of not smoking, your risk is similar to that of individuals who have never smoked.
>
> Five to fifteen years after you've stopped smoking, your chances of having a stroke are equal to that of people who have never smoked.
>
> After ten years without smoking, your risk of developing lung cancer declines to about one-half that of individuals who continue to smoke.

BECOMING A NON-SMOKER

Stopping smoking can be a life-saving decision. As a first step toward making cigarettes part of your past, take a few minutes to review the pros and cons of smoking by making some lists. On the 1st list, write down the most compelling reasons you want to stop smoking. You may want to quit for health reasons—perhaps to feel better and have more energy for daily activities. Or, you may want to decrease your risk of heart disease or cancer. Perhaps you want to be rid of a smoker's cough or eradicate excruciating angina (chest pain).

You might also feel that by stopping smoking you will serve as a better role model for your children, live long enough to become a grandparent, and spare those you live with from the health hazards of breathing second-hand smoke. Maybe you'd like to get rid of the tobacco odor in your home, the ashes and burn holes that mar your wardrobe, and the yellow stains on your teeth. Quitting will also save you a lot of money in cigarette costs, medical bills, and insurance premiums. Perhaps you've also concluded that smoking is fast becoming socially unacceptable in many circles.

LIST 1: I WANT TO STOP SMOKING BECAUSE: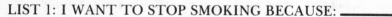

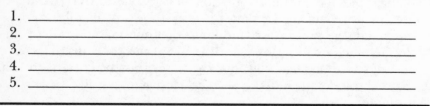

1. _____
2. _____
3. _____
4. _____
5. _____

On the next list, write down the most important reasons you want to continue smoking. In other words, what does smoking do for you? From your point of view, what needs does smoking meet? Maybe cigarettes help calm you down when you're feeling stressed. Smoking may provide you with a few moments of pleasure. It might make you feel more relaxed at social events, or help you stave off feelings of loneliness. It may give you something to do with your hands or help you concentrate during long hours of work. It may provide you with something to put in your mouth to curb your appetite and keep your weight under control.

LIST 2: I WANT TO CONTINUE SMOKING BECAUSE: _____

1. _____
2. _____
3. _____
4. _____
5. _____

Now, use your most creative brain-storming abilities to identify healthier ways of meeting the needs that smoking fulfills. For example, if you use cigarettes to relax and manage stress, substitute other methods to calm yourself, like the HART Program's techniques to deepen your breathing, relax your muscles, or warm your hands. If you find preferable ways to meet your needs, you will diminish the need to smoke until it withers and disappears. Rather than turning to a cigarette to combat loneliness, can you connect with a network of friends (preferably nonsmokers), join an organization, or take self-help classes in order to meet people? Can you more effectively manage your weight by using the nutritional information in this book, decreasing high-fat and high-sugar foods, and increasing fresh fruits and vegetables in your diet?

LIST 3: I CAN MEET MY SMOKING-RELATED NEEDS BY: ____

1. _____
2. _____
3. _____
4. _____
5. _____

Once you have filled in all three charts, evaluate the pros and cons of quitting and the preferred ways of meeting your needs. The next step is to begin using each urge to smoke as an opportunity to meet your needs in the preferable ways you have described.

KEEPING A DIARY

For the next few days, keep a log of your smoking habits. Each time you want a cigarette, jot down the time of day, the place, and what else you are doing (drinking coffee, talking on the phone) and feeling (fatigued, stressed).

You might discover that you smoke at your desk at work when you're feeling particularly anxious. Or that you reach for a cigarette whenever you pour yourself a cup of coffee. Or that you smoke after every meal, while you're driving in your car, or when you're bored.

Now that you have this information, you can begin to explore additional options for meeting the needs that cigarettes now fulfill. If smoking gives you self-confidence in social situations, maybe a new outfit or a new hairstyle will be even more effective. Instead of smoking to unwind or relax, use your CIP skills or go for a walk. Instead of putting a cigarette in your mouth, gnaw on a cinnamon stick, celery stalk, or even a pen. Expand upon your original list of ways to meet your needs without turning to cigarettes.

QUITTING THROUGH IMAGERY

There is another powerful tool that can help you quit smoking: the same type of relaxation and imagery exercises you may have used to implement stress management strategies or as an aid to weight loss.

Turn back to Chapter 12 to review how you can use imagery to change your behavior. By regularly imaging new preferred types of behavior, you will be able to implement them into your daily life more easily.

Plan on spending a few minutes each day—perhaps just after you wake up—picturing yourself engaging in behavior that will support you in living a smoke-free life. Make it a multisensory experience: not only see, but also feel and hear yourself choose healthier ways to meet the needs smoking fulfilled in the past.

For instance, picture yourself getting up after meals and taking a walk rather than lingering at the table with a cigarette. Visualize yourself feeling so much better as an ex-smoker; free of coughing and breathing problems, devoid of any nicotine cravings, and filled with so much more energy and enthusiasm for life. Imagine your lungs brimming with nourishing oxygen, rather than poisonous gases from cigarettes.

Picture a co-worker offering you a cigarette. Can you see yourself politely turning the offer down? Can you feel the satisfaction and the enhanced self-esteem that come with assertively saying no to smoking?

By using the imagery you develop at least once a day, you will mobilize important resources that will help you maintain a smoking-free lifestyle. On the positive side, if you have stopped and then started smoking again in the past, this will actually strengthen your likelihood of eventually stopping for good.

SELECTING A DAY TO QUIT

To strengthen your commitment to quit, choose a specific day to stop smoking for good. It should be a day when you expect to be relatively free of stress at work or at home.

The thought of going "cold turkey" scares some people; they'd prefer to taper off cigarettes gradually, decreasing their reliance on smoking a little at a time. However, people who cut back slowly often discover that the route can be less comfortable and less effective. A study published in the *Journal of the American Medical Association* in 1990 showed that smokers who quit "cold turkey" are more likely to quit for good than those who gradually taper off their use of cigarettes.

In those first few days of quitting, keep as busy as possible. If they are not work days, make sure you fill them with activities—long walks, bike rides, movies, and visits to nonsmoking friends. Prove to yourself that life can be enjoyable without cigarettes.

Stay away from cues that you associate with smoking, such as coffee or alcohol. Get plenty of exercise and rest. Ask for support from friends and relatives, particularly those who themselves have stopped smoking.

Incidentally, although you might experience some nicotine withdrawal symptoms—such as anxiety, irritability, restlessness, and difficulty concentrating—they are usually short-lived. They tend to peak in the first day or two, and then quickly become much less of a problem. Keep in mind that these uncomfortable symptoms are evidence that your body is successfully cleansing itself of nicotine. Breathe easier. You are about to start a new, healthier life.

WHAT IF YOU RELAPSE?

Many ex-smokers backslide several times before they finally quit for good. According to the Surgeon General, at least one-third of smokers who had stopped for a year or more may eventually experience a relapse.

However, don't let that statistic discourage you. As you stay off cigarettes for longer periods of time, your chances of another relapse decrease significantly.

If you do start smoking again, recognize that you've had a setback, and decide immediately to get back on track. Don't be too hard on yourself; instead, devote your energies toward returning to a smoke-free life. If possible, identify the trigger that prompted you to reach for a cigarette—perhaps a stress-producing deadline at work or an argument with your spouse. Make plans **now** to deal more constructively with the same situation the next time it arises—without resorting to cigarettes.

If you feel you need help, *The No-Nag, No-Guilt, Do-It-Your-Own-Way Guide to Quitting Smoking* by Tom Ferguson, M.D., is a superior resource. Free or low-cost stop-smoking programs are available from a number of organizations, such as the American Cancer Society and the American Heart Association. Nevertheless, about 90 percent of ex-smokers have quit on their own.

A final brief word about smoking: For the sake of your heart, blood vessels, and cardiovascular health, STOP!

CHAPTER 16

Commit To Be Cardiofit: Exercise for Lower Blood Pressure

Mens sana in corpore sano. (A sound mind in a sound body.)

—Latin proverb

All parts of the body which have a function, if used in moderation and exercised in labors in which each is accustomed, thereby become healthy, well-developed, and age more slowly; but if unused and left idle, they become liable to disease, defective in growth, and age quickly.

—HIPPOCRATES, 450 B.C.

GEORGE, A HART PROGRAM participant, may have been biologically predisposed to have high blood pressure. After all, both of his parents had hypertension and died of cardiovascular disease. His brother and one of his sisters also have elevated blood pressure. So when George's doctor diagnosed him as having hypertension, he wasn't completely surprised. Because his family health histories were so unsettling, George had a strong motivation to bring his own high blood pressure under control.

Despite George's busy schedule at work, he committed himself to regular relaxation, stress management, and other lifestyle changes—including physical exercise—that he thought could help him normalize his hypertension. Exercise played an important role in the control he eventually regained over his own blood pressure and well-being. "I started to swim, and I was amazed at what that did for my blood pressure," George recalls. "Even though I'm not a great swimmer, the physical exertion in the water was very good for me."

George found still other ways to incorporate exercise into his life. He now walks to and from work every day—a three-mile roundtrip—and relies on public transportation only when the weather is particularly bad. He also bought a rowing machine that has become part of his exercise program to make sure his upper body stays strong.

George has found that when his weight creeps up, so does his blood pressure. The added exercise is not only helping him normalize his blood pressure, it is also helping him control his weight, while allowing him to fulfill his goal of being cardiofit for life.

Gary, another patient in the HART Program, began exercising as well—but not without some unexpected turns of events. He found that the beta-blocker medication he was taking kept his heart rate so low during exercise that he wasn't getting much of a cardiovascular workout. However, as his blood pressure came down through relaxation and stress management—and, in turn, as his doctor was able to reduce the dosage of his medication and then eventually eliminate it—his resting pulse rate was no longer being kept low by the drugs. In fact, his pulse rate was suddenly **higher** than desirable! Because Gary knew that a higher pulse rate can contribute to higher blood pressure, he worked toward the additional goal of bringing his resting pulse rate down.

Gary continued with his exercise, relaxation, and stress management practice, and soon his heart rate declined. When it did, he gradually increased the duration of his aerobic exercise sessions, using the treadmill and other equipment at his health club. Through these regular workouts, he was able to train in his target heart rate zone and regain a slower, healthier, athletic pulse—and lower blood pressure.

Julia always swam regularly as part of her personal program to manage her blood pressure. She swam before starting the HART Program, but that isn't the only exercise she gets now. Seeing the positive effect swimming had on her blood pressure, Julia decided to increase her exercise by walking or biking to and from the pool. Between her regular relaxation and stress management practice and exercise, not only is Julia's blood pressure under control, but her cholesterol levels have returned to normal.

HOW IMPORTANT IS EXERCISE?

The human body was built to move. Until recently, however, most doctors didn't take exercise seriously—especially for patients with heart problems. In fact, if you had hypertension and other cardiovascular diseases, exercise was probably off-limits if you followed your doctor's orders.

In the late nineteenth century, a book for physicians advised that patients in the early stages of heart disease avoid "all causes of exertion." These sentiments were echoed in 1927 in a well-known medical volume, *Cecil's A Textbook of Medicine*, which recommended that people with heart disorders and hypertension "avoid all overtaxation of the heart." That's the way most hypertensives were treated until the late 1950s.

But times have changed. Today, your doctor is as likely to encourage you to exercise as to reach for a pen to write a prescription for antihypertensive drugs. And much of the credit for that goes to pioneers like cardiologist Paul Dudley White. In observing his own patients, Dr. White began to recognize that getting out of their easy chairs and putting their bodies into motion could have significant benefits. Too many patients with heart disease, he noticed, were being needlessly turned into invalids, and as a result, their health was undermined.

Dr. White became an outspoken champion of physical fitness. When President Dwight Eisenhower suffered a heart attack in 1955, Dr. White encouraged him to return to the golf course after a period of convalescence. He wrote: "Exercise to keep fit . . . . To have good muscles and a freely moving diaphragm, not obstructed by abdominal fat, is an important and vital element in maintaining good health and in aiding the heart and blood vessels in their work."

Since then, tens of thousands of doctors have become convinced of the merits of regular exercise in lowering blood pressure and maintaining cardiovascular health. Your own cardiologist has probably told you that moderately-vigorous exercise—such as brisk walking or bicycling—will not only help lower your blood pressure and protect against heart attacks and strokes, it is also an excellent way to transform your heart and vasculature into a more efficient life-support system. Like any muscle, the heart becomes stronger and more efficient the more it is used, allowing it to pump more oxygen-rich blood with each beat. At the same time, your heart will beat more slowly and the entire circulatory system will work with less fatigue—and with minimal increases in blood pressure during periods of exertion. While the resting heart rate of the average sedentary person may be 70 to 80 beats per minute and that of a well-conditioned exerciser 65 beats, long-distance runners often have pulse rates as low as 40 to 50 beats a minute—or even less. The slower the heart beat, the greater the flow of blood through the coronary arteries and into the heart, since blood actually enters the heart's chambers only **between** beats.

Also, according to some studies, vigorous or aerobic exercise stimulates the growth of new capillaries branching off the coronary arteries—a phenomenon that may decrease the chances of a heart attack by providing alternate routes for blood if the main pathways become clogged. In a sense, this "collateral circulation" creates a natural heart bypass. In the process, as your circulating blood encounters less resistance and your heart is forced to work less vigorously, your blood pressure will tend to decline as your chances of having a coronary or a stroke also decrease. More specifically, aerobic exercise requires increased oxygen use over an extended time period (minimally fifteen minutes), and involves the continuous movement of large muscles that can speed up the flow of blood to the heart. With these exercises, individuals can work out in their target heart zone, a range required to achieve cardiovascular fitness.

Not surprisingly, then, regular physical activity is important not only in reducing your blood pressure, but also in protecting your overall cardiovascular health. To maximize your chances of normalizing your blood pressure, regular exercise is essential. Find time for a fitness program, no matter what your age.

How strong is the evidence linking exercise with declines in blood pressure? Keep in mind that most studies show that if you have mild to moderate hypertension, exercise can reduce your blood pressure readings by between 5 and 15 mmHg. When you combine physical activity with the other components of the HART Program—especially, relaxation, stress management and a high complex-carbohydrate, low-fat diet—your blood pressure should decrease even more significantly.

There is another important advantage to physical activity. A regular, vigorous program of exercise adds balance and resilience to your life. Individuals who exercise regularly tend to manage stress more efficiently and resist illness better, whether it is the common cold or serious cardiovascular disease. They just plain feel better. So, although relaxation is a core component of the HART Program, exercise is just as important; it helps you achieve some of relaxation's objectives, from burning up stress hormones to reducing your resting heart rate.

OUR SEDENTARY LIVES

In earlier generations, most people didn't have to worry about getting enough exercise. They expended considerable amounts of energy on the job, getting from place to place, and keeping their households running. However, the industrial revolution changed all that. In the workplace, machines replaced strenuous human labor. At home, most people acquired labor-saving appliances and their automobiles rarely forced them to break into a sweat.

If anything, the trend toward a sedentary life is more pronounced than ever. If you're like many people, you drive to work in your car or take public transportation, ride an elevator up to your office, sit behind a desk for eight hours, then return home to a microwave-cooked dinner and an evening of watching television. It is hard to imagine a more passive—and perhaps self-destructive—way to live.

Nevertheless, too many Americans seem hopelessly attached to inactivity. Only about 20 percent of the adult population exercise vigorously and often enough to gain cardiovascular benefits. When people are sedentary, they are just setting themselves up for health problems, since they are more prone to hypertension, heart attacks, obesity, osteoporosis, and depression.

Activity is a basic physiological requirement; it is actually abnormal not to be in motion for at least 20 minutes a day. People who don't get their bodies in motion may pay the price with their health. Just remember: **it is never too late to start an exercise program.** As you read this chapter, you will discover that for the relatively small amount of time and effort you invest in exercise, your health and well-being will reap enormous benefits, including the slowing of the aging process. People who exercise regularly tend to be biologically younger than their chronological age and their sedentary peers.

If you have not exercised in years, however, don't despair. According to Steven Blair, director of epidemiology at the Institute for Aerobics Research, research indicates that the greatest benefits from exercise are achieved by people whose degree of fitness is the lowest. He adds that you are better off doing anything rather than nothing, particularly if you have not exercised at all in recent months. Begin with short walks, recreational sports or gardening. Slowly increase your activity, allowing your body to be your guide.

EXERCISE & YOUR HEART

Several years ago, Dr. Ralph Paffenbarger of Stanford University set out to quantify the effect that physical activity has on human health by studying approximately 15,000 male alumni of Harvard University. He found that individuals participating in strenuous sports—for example, swimming, running, handball, or basketball—had fewer heart attacks and other "cardiac events." Less intense activities, such as bowling or golf, did not have the same protective effect.

According to Dr. Paffenbarger, people expending 2,000 calories a week through exercise had a heart attack rate approximately half that of individuals who only used up 500 calories a week during physical activity. The study also showed that when people did not make vigorous exercise part of their lives, they had a 35 percent higher chance of developing hypertension, whether or not they were obese or had a family history of high blood pressure.

In his 1986 followup report, Dr. Paffenbarger continued to see a similar trend. Death rates, he concluded, were "significantly lower among the physically active."

A chorus of other studies substantiates the benefits of exercise:

Researchers at the Cooper Clinic in Dallas examined the exercise habits and the health status of 6,039 men and women who had normal blood pressure readings when the study began. Over the ensuing 12 years, the participants with poor physical fitness had a 52 percent greater chance of developing hypertension than those who were more fit.

In the Chicago Coronary Prevention Evaluation program, subjects exercised at least three times a week, while simultaneously reducing their caloric consumption by 30 percent. Most patients lost weight and experienced reductions in their blood pressure readings. Among 67 middle-aged hypertensives who were not taking drugs for their high blood pressure, systolic pressures declined an average of 13.3 mm Hg, and diastolic readings fell an average of 9.7 mm Hg.

Dr. Robert Cade headed up a study at the University of Florida involving 105 hypertensive patients (ages 22 to 66), all of whom began the study with diastolic blood pressure exceeding 90 mm Hg. Slightly less than half of them were taking antihypertensive medication. All participants began a vigorous exercise program, beginning with a one-mile walk each day, and eventually progressing to a two-mile daily jog. Within three months after reaching the two-mile plateau, 96 percent of the participants had experienced significant declines in their blood pressure readings. About half of those who had been taking drugs were able to discontinue using them, thanks to an average decline in diastolic pressure from 116.9 to 97.2 mm Hg.

At the Veterans Administration Medical Center in Jackson, Mississippi, adult males with mild hypertension adopted an exercise program four days a week. Their physical activity consisted of 30 minutes of either brisk walking/jogging or pedaling a stationary bicycle. After ten weeks, their systolic blood pressure had declined an average of 13.7 mm Hg, while their diastolic readings had dipped an average of 9.7 mm Hg. A later study by the same researchers recorded decreases in diastolic readings averaging 9.6 mm Hg in hypertensive patients who exercised, compared to a 0.8 mm Hg **increase** in the non-exercising hypertensives.

OTHER BENEFITS: WHAT ELSE CAN EXERCISE DO?

By now, you should be seeing the strong rationale for making exercise a regular part of your life. Once you've adopted a fitness program, particularly if you are not already exercising, you will find that there is even more to be gained from physical activity than "just" its positive effect on your blood pressure. Here are some of the other benefits you can expect:

1. **Alleviation of Stress.** Regular exercise, like relaxation and stress management, helps "inoculate" you against the more harmful effects of stress. It is a natural way to deal with the pressures and anxieties of life, helping you achieve a healthy balance without resorting to alcohol, drugs, or other potentially-harmful substances. In fact, adults who exercise regularly tend to drink considerably less alcohol than those who don't; children who exercise tend to use far fewer drugs than their sedentary contemporaries.

   When your body is in a fight-or-flight condition, exercise is an efficient way to turn off that aroused state. At Duke University, researchers found that when Type A (compulsive, easily angered, hard-driving personality) individuals participated in a walking/jogging program (three miles per day, three days a week), their Type A characteristics became less dominant in their lives.

   Physical activity fights stress another way: exercise can result in a slower resting heart rate, which can keep you more relaxed and in control during stressful periods. Also, if you exercise near the end of the day—right after work, for example—there's some evidence that you will burn up secreted stress hormones like adrenaline that build up during the morning and afternoon. This will leave you in a state of greater equilibrium for the evening hours. People relax more easily after exercising; in fact, regular exercise is a natural complement to your deep relaxation practice.

2. **Improved Sleep Habits.** Exercise enhances the quality of your sleep. In addition to leaving you refreshed, sound sleep is an important buffer against stress. When deprived of adequate sleep, some individuals tend to have higher blood pressure. Most people require seven to eight hours of sleep at night for good health and longevity.

3. **Enhanced "Vital Capacity."** Since your vital capacity, or lung capacity, is an important predictor of longevity, it makes sense to increase it. As we age, our ability to utilize large amounts of oxygen declines. Nothing can counteract that process better than physical activity in tandem with the deep diaphragmatic breathing technique you learned earlier in the book. If you exercise regularly and don't smoke, you are more likely to have the oxygen capacity of someone at least a decade or two younger. A 70-year-old person who exercises routinely may

have the same vital capacity as a non-exercising 20-year-old. An active lifestyle can also fortify the muscles involved in breathing, making diaphragmatic breathing more effortless, at rest, as well as during strenuous activities.

4. **Natural Endorphin Highs.** As you exercise, chemicals called endorphins are released into your bloodstream. These endorphins are natural mood elevators, and are probably responsible for the "runner's high" that some joggers describe, and the natural exhilaration that many people feel when engaging in the aerobic exercise of their choice. Some research has shown that the more regularly you exercise, the more rapidly your endorphins rise after you've started working out—and the longer they stay elevated after you stop moving. Many people claim they're "addicted" to exercise—a healthy addiction, to be sure—feeling great when they are physically active. Endorphins may deserve the credit.

5. **Eased Depression: Improved Outlook.** Other chemicals in the body associated with mood are also influenced by exercise; specifically, norepinephrine, serotonin, and dopamine. These substances, which transmit messages between nerves, tend to be deficient in depressed individuals. However, during exercise, they are secreted into the brain in larger amounts, easing depression in the process.

A number of studies support an association between exercise and an elevated mood. At the National Institute of Health, recent research involving 1,900 men and women showed that moderate exercise could reduce by half the risk of developing depressive symptoms ranging from crying spells to a lack of enjoyment of life. Another study at Purdue University, in which 58 men participated in an exercise program consisting of jogging, calisthenics, and recreational activities, reported an increase in self-confidence and signs of greater emotional stability due to exercise.

6. **Increased Energy and Stamina.** Because you expend a lot of energy when you're active, common sense might suggest that exercise depletes your energy. In reality, once your body has adapted to a regular exercise regime, the opposite is true: physical activity makes you **more** energetic and refreshed. People who exercise regularly have more stamina throughout the day than their sedentary peers.

7. **Weight Management.** Physical activity can help normalize your weight in a number of ways. For example, while occasional exercise can increase your appetite, a regular fitness program tends to have the opposite effect; it actually decreases your

desire for food. It can also raise your metabolic rate, thus increasing the expenditure of calories even after you've stopped exercising. In addition to burning calories and fat, exercise firms and tones your body, replacing fat with lean muscle. Since most calories are burned by lean body mass (or muscle), the more lean muscle you have, the quicker you will shed excess weight and the more likely you will be to keep it off.

HOW MANY CALORIES DO YOU BURN DURING EXERCISE?

Exercise	Calories Expended Per Hour
Walking (4.5 mph)	400
Tennis (moderate level)	425
Swimming	530
Handball	600
Jogging (5.5 mph)	650
Bicycling (13 mph)	850

---

8. **Decreased Platelet Aggregation.** There is more good news about physical activity and your cardiovascular system. Exercise minimizes the tendency of platelets in your blood to stick to one another. These small structures, which help keep blood coagulation normal, can also cause the formation of blood clots if they cling together. With even moderate exercise, however, you can reduce the chances of platelets playing a role in provoking a heart attack.

9. **Stronger Bones.** As people grow older, they become increasingly vulnerable to *osteoporosis,* a disorder that involves thinning of the bones. Twenty million Americans suffer from osteoporosis: about 30 percent of women and 10 percent of men over 60 have this condition, and beyond the age of 70, about 50 percent of people have it. Over the years, bones tend to become more brittle and increasingly susceptible to breaking—even during everyday motions like stepping off a curb. Postmenopausal women are particularly vulnerable to this disorder since they can no longer count on natural estrogen hormones to keep their bones strong and thick.

    Osteoporosis is not inevitable, however. Participating in weight-bearing exercise, such as running, walking, low-impact aerobic dance, resistance training with light weights, or stairclimbing, while also keeping your calcium and magnesium consumption high, can help prevent this disorder. An active lifestyle actually retards the loss of bone mass, and as your bones maintain their strength—or even become stronger—you will become less prone to fractures, which can be life-threatening in the later years. All bodies, regardless of their age, respond to strengthening programs.

10. **Better Cholesterol Levels: Higher HDL, Lower LDL.** As you'll recall from Chapter 12, there are two types of cholesterol in your bloodstream: LDL (low-density lipoprotein) and HDL (high-density lipoprotein). While your LDL needs to be kept as low as possible, this is not the case with HDL. After all, HDL is the "good" cholesterol, which protects against heart disease by removing plaque-forming fats from the bloodstream. Thus, the higher your HDL, the lower your risk of heart problems.

How does exercise fit into this picture? Studies indicate that when men and women exercise regularly and vigorously, their HDL levels tend to increase. And that's exactly the effect you want to keep your heart and vascular system healthy.

DIFFERENT KINDS OF EXERCISE

As you have seen, exercise can play an important role not only in reducing your blood pressure, but in enhancing many other aspects of your physical and mental well-being. If you have been exercising regularly, you may already know this from your own experience. If you aren't yet physically active, it's time to get started with your own fitness program.

As you begin, keep in mind that the **kind** of exercise you select is extremely important. There are two broad categories from which to choose: aerobic and anaerobic exercise.

AEROBIC EXERCISE

If you have hypertension or other cardiovascular health problems, aerobic exercise will give you the greatest cardiovascular benefit. Aerobic activity can help get your heart and vasculature into shape, and keep them that way. By definition, aerobic means "with oxygen." It involves vigorously working the body's large-muscle groups, particularly the legs and arms, for a sustained period of time (a minimum of fifteen minutes), which sets off a chain reaction of positive bodily processes. First, the heart and breathing rates accelerate, causing the flow of blood and oxygen to every part of the body to increase dramatically. Whereas the heart pumps about 6 quarts of blood a minute in a typical non-exercising individual, this rises to about 25 quarts per minute during aerobic activity. Over time, this strengthens the muscles and increases the body's network of blood vessels.

What are the best types of aerobic exercise? Brisk walking, running, jogging, swimming, and bicycling are excellent aerobic activities. No matter which you choose, by gradually increasing the duration, intensity, and frequency of your aerobic activity, you will experience a rapid build-up of stamina. For instance, while you may be able to walk or jog for only a few minutes when you begin, with perseverance, you will soon find yourself able to walk or run for a half-hour or more.

ANAEROBIC EXERCISE

This type of exercise involves movements of only brief intensity, followed by relatively lengthy periods of inactivity. As a result, there is not the same sustained supply of oxygen to the muscles. Anaerobic ("without oxygen") activities include weight-lifting, golf, bowling, baseball, and doubles tennis. Of course, anaerobic exercise is not completely without oxygen use, but it does not require the same high level of oxygen as exercise classified as aerobic. You may find that weight training tones your muscles and that golf, tennis, or other sports are socially enjoyable; however, they won't provide you with the sustained movement that's required to build and maintain your cardiovascular fitness. You'd be wise to adopt an aerobic type of exercise as well.

A word of caution, however: If you have hypertension, you may need to avoid exercises like heavy weight-lifting or other so-called *isometric* exercises, in which muscles contract against resistance. When lifting heavy weights, both your systolic and diastolic blood pressure can rise excessively, which could create serious strain upon your heart. However, one recent study indicates that circuit training with **light** weights can be beneficial in lowering blood pressure. Consult your doctor and exercise physiologist before beginning any exercise program. The risks associated with isometrics can also occur in everyday activities such as shoveling snow, picking up a heavy suitcase, or opening a stuck window—so think before you lift, or if so advised by your doctor, delegate lifting responsibilities to someone else.

Aerobic Exercises

Brisk walking	Cross-country skiing
Running/jogging	Roller skating
Swimming	Ice skating
Aerobic dancing	Rowing
Bicycle riding	Jumping rope
Stationary cycling	Soccer

Anaerobic Exercises

Golf	Football
Bowling	Racketball*
Sprinting	Tennis*
Weight-lifting	Handball*
Baseball	

* If performed at a high intensity with nearly continuous motion for fifteen minutes or more within your target heart rate zone, these exercises can qualify as aerobic.

CHOOSING THE BEST EXERCISE FOR YOU

What aerobic activities are best for you? This section briefly describes some of the more popular alternatives. No matter what exercise you choose, keep one thing in mind: **Exercise is best if it's fun.** The one you enjoy is probably the best exercise for you. By selecting an aerobic exercise you enjoy—or, even better, by cultivating two or three forms of exercise to vary the activity of your muscle groups and keep your interest high—you will look forward to exercise and make time for an aerobic program in your schedule.

BRISK WALKING

Along with swimming and jogging, walking has become one of our nation's most popular aerobic activities. No matter what your age or fitness level, you can walk—even if you are overweight, suffer from arthritis, have experienced a heart attack, or have undergone bypass surgery. (Particularly in the latter two cases, you should be under a doctor's care, and following his or her recommendations about when to start exercising and whether you should be in a supervised, rehabilitative exercise program.) You don't need to invest any money in equipment, except for a good pair of walking shoes—an investment well worth making. You can walk almost anywhere.

There is another important advantage to brisk walking: It is a relatively risk-free activity. Compared to jogging, walking causes very few injuries, primarily because it doesn't expose the body to percussive jolts.

However, walking as an aerobic exercise means **brisk** walking, rather than just a leisurely saunter. You will need to adopt a stride that is longer than normal, keeping your back straight and relaxed, with your arms swinging at your sides. Land on your heels, point your toes straight ahead, and push off on the balls of your feet.

Like many other people, you may wonder if brisk walking is really as beneficial as more strenuous activities—will it help control your high blood pressure as effectively as jogging? Recent research at the Washington University School of Medicine concluded that it can. In that study, 33 hypertensive patients (average age—64) were placed in one of three groups: some adopted a walking program (one hour, three times a week); others began with walking, but gradually escalated into more intense activity, including jogging and stationary cycling (45 to 60 minutes, three times a week); the final group did not exercise at all.

Both the walking and jogging groups experienced nearly identical declines in diastolic blood pressure—11 to 12 mm Hg—after several months of exercise. But there was an even more surprising finding. Systolic pressure declined 20 mm Hg in the walking group, which was significantly **greater** than the systolic decreases experienced by the higher-intensity exercisers. "Thus," the researchers concluded, "low-intensity training may lower blood pressure as much or more than moderate-intensity training in older persons with essential hypertension."

If you jog, like it, and have your physician's approval, stay with it. For many people, brisk walking may be just what the doctor ordered.

JOGGING/RUNNING

Jogging and running provide an excellent aerobic workout, which can help control both weight and hypertension.

Unfortunately, jogging places more stress on your joints and muscles than walking. Even so, by running the proper way, you can cut down your risk of injury. As you run, land on your heels and push off with your toes; if you run only on your toes, you will increase the strain on your knees. When you land, your foot should be directly beneath your knee.

Some people find grass an ideal surface for running, although because many grassy areas have uneven terrain and divots, you need to exercise more care to prevent twisting injuries of the ankles or knees. Instead, you may want to look for a resilient running track at a local high school or community park. If you decide to run on asphalt or cement, be sure to wear a good pair of running shoes.

BICYCLING

Bicycling is an especially good alternative to jogging if you have an orthopedic problem like a bad back or knee. For outdoor cycling, begin your exercise program on level ground with the bicycle's gears at the lowest setting. During the upcoming weeks, as you build up strength and endurance, gradually shift to higher gears and add some inclines to your exercise course. And for safety, wear a bicycle helmet at all times.

You can also choose a stationary bicycle for your exercise program. This will permit you to work out even in inclement weather—while avoiding traffic hazards at the same time. Most stationary bicycles have calibrated knobs that allow you to raise and lower the pedal tension so you can simulate going uphill. For a good aerobic workout, change the tension periodically, lowering it as you become tired, then raising it again as your energy returns.

SWIMMING

According to the President's Council on Physical Fitness and Sports, swimming has more participants than any other sport. Swimming provides a workout for the entire body, not just the cardiovascular system.

When you swim, concentrate on your favorite stroke, or vary from one stroke to another to avoid boredom. In most strokes, like the crawl and the backstroke, keep your legs nearly straight as you kick, creating most of the power in your hips.

Don't ignore safety when you swim. If you feel yourself becoming fatigued, rest for a few minutes. Whenever possible, swim with a friend or a lifeguard nearby. During dips in the ocean or a lake, swim parallel to the shore so you can reach land quickly if you become tired.

LOW-IMPACT AEROBIC DANCING

If you enjoy group energy, strong leadership, and moving to music, then low-impact aerobic dancing may be for you. It is a wonderful way to increase your fitness and endurance while having fun at the same time.

When choosing an aerobic dance class, find a teacher you like and a program that meets your exercise needs. I strongly urge you to choose a **low-impact** aerobics program, now offered at many health clubs. Low-impact programs are choreographed to use your large body muscles **without** the jumping you would find in high-impact aerobics. Leaving out the jumping and bouncing significantly reduces your chances of injury.

In a single exercise session, a good aerobic dance class will be combined with a warm-up period, an aerobics session (at least 25 to 45 minutes of vigorous exercise), a cooldown time, stretching, and in some cases, even some muscle toning. Be sure you wear a good pair of aerobic shoes. Try to find a class in which you will be exercising on resilient wooden floors. As you become increasingly fit, you may wish to find low-impact classes that also use light (one- or two-pound) weights on each wrist to give your upper body a workout and help keep your pulse rate up.

GETTING OUT OF THE STARTING BLOCKS

Before HART Program participants begin exercising, they are strongly advised to see their physician. **You should see your doctor, too.** This is particularly important if you have high blood pressure, are over the age of 35, have a personal or family history or cardiovascular disease, are overweight, have high cholesterol, or are a heavy cigarette smoker. Have a physical exam and any tests that your doctor recommends, including an exercise stress test that monitors your cardiac activity and blood pressure during physical exertion (walking on a treadmill). The results will help you and your doctor and/or exercise physiologist create an exercise program specifically for you, taking into account your high blood pressure and other cardiovascular disorders. With this information in hand, you will have the peace of mind of knowing that you can exercise safely.

In addition to your doctor's recommendations, here are some points that are integral to implementing your personal cardiofitness program:

1. **Don't be in a hurry.** When it comes to exercise, some people want to do too much, too soon. This is a risky approach to exercise. There's no truth to the maxim, "No Pain, No Gain." In fact, exercise should be pain-free.

   In your first few sessions, start out slowly, particularly if you have been leading a sedentary lifestyle. Map out the initial distance you want to walk, jog, or bicycle, using the odometer on your car (or a pedometer). Plan on staying in motion for at least fifteen minutes in your first few sessions. Then, over time, gradually increase your pace, the distance you cover, and the length of your exercise routine. Your body requires time to adapt to increased exercise or to a change in the type of physical activity. Eventually, you will progress to 30 or more minutes of exercise per session. Many HART patients exercise for 45 minutes, one hour, or even longer.
2. **Exercise at least four to six times a week.** Aerobics pioneer and expert Dr. Kenneth Cooper recommends that you exercise no less than three times a week. Many individuals fare much better—in terms of physical and psychological benefits—when they exercise four, five, and even six times weekly. Although some people like to exercise seven days a week, you might profit

from a day off, allowing your body to rest and giving tired muscles or joints a chance to recuperate.

Incidentally, it is best not to be only a weekend or a "now-and-then" athlete. If you are, you might be asking for trouble. The body "detrains" very quickly, and by exercising only once in a while, you may never become strong enough to withstand a really vigorous workout. Exercise needs to become a regular habit you enjoy and can't live without.

3. **Incorporate warmup and cooldown periods into your exercise program.** Imagine the shock your body would feel if you stepped out your front door and immediately raised your heart rate from a resting level of about 75 beats a minute to 165 beats. Just like a car that needs a few minutes to warm up, your heart and circulatory system require some time to adjust to an accelerated level of physical activity.

Thus, no matter what form of exercise you choose, be kind to your body and spend at least five minutes warming up before the strenuous portion of your activity begins. That means starting with a slower, easier version of the same exercise that you've selected, which will permit blood to nourish those muscles that are about to be used. If you've chosen brisk walking as your exercise, the warm-up period should consist of a few minutes of relaxed, unhurried walking, during which you gradually build up to a more rapid pace.

In much the same way, make sure you cool down for three to five minutes after the intense phase of your exercise period. This generally consists of continued but less vigorous movement. If you're walking, slow down your pace; if you're running, downshift into a very slow jog, followed by a few minutes of walking.

If you don't take time to cool down, too much blood might remain in the muscles you used during exercise, such as your legs, rather than returning to your central circulatory system. That might leave your brain and heart short of blood, causing light-headedness, dizziness, and perhaps even more serious problems. The cool down also allows your blood pressure to subside, and heat production to decline.

4. **Add stretching and strengthening.** Balance your aerobics with a few minutes of stretching and strengthening exercises to maintain flexibility and keep your muscles well-conditioned and toned. Both are important to your overall fitness.

Without regular stretching, many people find their muscles become extraordinarily tight. Stretching can also prevent soreness and injuries related to your overall exercise program. Make sure you do your stretching slowly, without the jerking or bouncing that can actually cause muscles to contract reflexively, and thus tighten them even further. Many fitness experts now recommend that you do your stretching at the end of your aerobic exercise period to help keep your muscles from becoming tight.

If you use weights as part of your strengthening exercises, use only **light** weights. Isometric movements with heavy weights should be avoided by hypertensive patients. Keep the weights light and gradually increase the repetitions to make your workout more challenging.

For more specific information on developing your own aerobic exercise and stretching and strengthening program, consult *The Aerobics Way* or *The Aerobics Program for Total Well-being* by Kenneth Cooper, M.D. The Canadian Royal Exercise Program also offers a time-efficient set of exercises.

In addition, hatha yoga provides excellent methods of stretching and tuning both body and mind. In this area, consult *Integral Yoga Hatha* by Swami Satchidananda, *The Complete Illustrated Book of Yoga,* by Swami Vishnudevananda, and *Light on Yoga* by BKS Iyengar.

5. **Select and write down your exercise goals.** Do you plan to walk for fifteen minutes a day—Monday, Wednesday, Friday, and Saturday—for the first two weeks of your program, then escalate up to 25 minutes a day for the following two weeks, then to 40 minutes thereafter? No matter what your goals are, write them down in an exercise diary. You are more likely to stick to your program if you put it in writing and if your goals are realistic and achievable.

6. **Ask your doctor how medication could affect your exercise program.** Most drugs won't preclude you from exercising, but they may cause side effects that can influence your physical activity. These side effects must be considered when you're planning an exercise regimen. Diuretics, for example, can cause symptoms ranging from dehydration to arrhythmias. Beta-blockers have been associated with fatigue and may interfere with exercise-induced increases in heart rate, thus limiting the benefits you get from the program. If you are taking betablockers you also may need to be careful about avoiding overexertion, since the drug makes your pulse rate an inaccurate monitor of fatigue. In this case, pay close attention to your own subjective sense of how fatigued you are, and your perceived level of exertion.

Your commitment to exercise could influence your doctor's choice of antihypertensive and other types of medication. Regular aerobic activity may also decrease your need for medication as your blood pressure declines. Let your physician know about your physical activity; if your doctor knows that you are taking charge of your health and, when possible, want to eliminate your need for medication, he or she will be better able to support you in these goals.

7. **If you exercise outdoors, have a backup indoor activity planned for rainy, snowy, exceedingly cold, hot, humid, or highly-polluted days.** When walking or jogging becomes impractical because of weather conditions, have an alternative aerobic plan ready. Take out your jump rope, climb aboard a stationary bicycle, or head for the indoor swimming pool or exercise class at your local health club. Don't let the elements interfere with your exercise goals. As a general rule for cold weather exercising, exercise indoors whenever the outdoor windchill index dips below 15 degrees Farhenheit.

HOW MUCH IS TOO MUCH?

If you're exercising too hard, your body has its own way of telling you. Pay particular attention to the following signals:

If you feel faint, dizzy or nauseous—or if you experience pain or tightness in your chest, unusual heart rhythms, palpitations, severe shortness of breath, or loss of muscle control—**stop exercising immediately** and contact your doctor.

Five minutes after you've finished exercising, count your pulse. If it is 120 beats per minute or more, you are overdoing it. The same is true if your pulse rate is 100 or more, 10 minutes after you've stopped exercising. The next time you work out, ease up a bit on the intensity.

How's your breathing? Ten minutes after exercising, you should no longer be short of breath. If you are, you're overdoing it.

Exercise should be invigorating, not totally fatiguing. If you're worn out and exhausted for hours after your workout, even following a period of rest, you need to cut back on the intensity and build up your endurance more gradually.

FINDING YOUR TARGET HEART RATE

Exercise can become so enjoyable that sometimes you might feel that you could walk or run faster and farther than ever before. This can be an exhilarating experience if you have built up to a higher intensity level through regular training and you're staying within what is technically referred to as your *target heart zone.*

Keep in mind, however, that it is possible to exercise **too** strenuously, often without even realizing it. To prevent this, you need to find and work within your ideal training zone or target heart rate. This zone will help you exercise in a safe range, achieving cardiovascular conditioning without placing yourself at risk.

FINDING YOUR TARGET HEART RATE

Your target heart rate is approximately 60 to 90 percent of your **maximum** heart rate. Although a stress test can precisely pinpoint this figure, here's one formula to help you calculate it on your own. This method (the Karnoven method) is the one used by many members of the American College of Sports Medicine, as well as the International Dance and Exercise Association.

1. Take the number 210 (for women) or 220 (for men), and subtract your entire age if you are female and half your age if you are male. This figure is your maximum heart rate.
2. Subtract your resting rate.*

   Two samples of this calculation appear in the box on the following page.

   Once you know your target heart rate, you need to learn to count your pulse while exercising. Many people find it easiest to place their fingers on either side of the neck, locating the pulse below the jaw and alongside the windpipe. You can also use the pulse at your wrist. While you are exercising, stop for a moment, quickly locate your pulse and count the number of heart beats for ten seconds, using the second hand on your watch as a timer. For accuracy, start your first count at zero. Multiply this number by six—this will give you the number of heart beats per minute.** If this number exceeds your target heart rate, taper off your exercise a little bit; if it's lower than your target zone, increase your intensity.

---

*To find your resting heart rate, locate the pulse point at your wrist or on your neck near the throat. Apply light, firm pressure with your fingers. Count the number of beats over a 30-second period, and then multiply by 2. That is your resting heart rate.

** This is a shorter monitoring interval (10 seconds) than we used to determine your resting heart rate (30 seconds). It will allow you to obtain a reading before your pulse decelerates during your aerobic exercise period.

3. To determine your ideal exercising zone, multiply that answer by .60 and .90 and then add your resting heart rate to each of these numbers.

Calculating Your Target Heart Rate: Two Examples

Women				*Men*	
220				210	
− 40	(age)			− 20	(½ age)
180		(maximum heart rate)		190	
− 70		(resting heart rate)		− 70	
110	110			120	120
× .60	× .90			× .60	× .90
66	99			72	108
+ 70	+ 70	(resting heart rate)		+ 70	+ 70
137	169			142	178

In these examples, the woman's heart rate should fall between 137 and 169 beats per minute while exercising, while the man's heart rate should fall in the 142 to 178 range.

To optimize the cardiovascular benefits of your aerobics activity, get into your target heart range after your warm-up, staying between 60 and 90 percent of your maximum heart rate throughout the aerobic phase of your exercise. When you're just beginning an exercise program, keep your heart beating near the lower end of your target range; over a period of weeks, gradually work your way up to the higher end of the spectrum.

However, be sure to ask your doctor for specific guidance that is appropriate just for you. Depending on your physical condition, your doctor may recommend that you not exceed 75 percent of your maximum heart rate—or perhaps even less in some cases. Follow the advice of your own physician closely.

It is also advisable to become sensitive to your own "perceived exertion level," a concept created by Swedish researchers as a way to monitor one's own exercise intensity. It is based on the theory that over time, we can all begin to sense when we're exercising too strenuously—or not strenuously enough. In general, if you're gasping for breath, you're overdoing it; while if you're not breathing much above your resting rate, you need to pick up the pace.

STICKING WITH IT

Everyone experiences days when they just don't feel like exercising. Yes, you understand the importance of physical activity; at times, however, you just feel too tired, too depressed, or too busy. Maybe you're feeling stiff or you're beginning to find exercise "boring."

On days like these, it sometimes helps to pick yourself up and go to the place where you exercise—a running track or health club—and start your activity. Only make the decision whether to continue exercising once your endorphin levels have risen during those first few minutes of your workout. Don't let excuses and obstacles get the better of you.

Constructive self-talk can be very useful here. Acknowledge your inner state ("Yes, I'm feeling tired today"), but remind yourself that you'll feel better if you move ("I'm going to exercise because I know my tired feelings will disappear once I'm in motion").

Quite frankly, your blood pressure and overall health are too important to ignore exercise. Everyone runs into barriers, but there are ways to break through them. Here are some other suggestions:

If boredom is setting in, find some way to vary your environment, your exercise, or your thoughts during your sessions. For example, if walking, running, or bicycling is the mainstay of your exercise program, alter your route. A change of scenery may be all you need. Using a pedometer or the odometer of your car, calculate the distance of your new exercise course so you can stick to your regimen of one, two, or three miles.

If you are tired, breathe more deeply and repeat internally, "The more I move (run, walk), the more energized I feel."

Combine exercise with an activity you find enjoyable. For instance, buy yourself a cassette player with headphones and let your favorite music accompany your exercising or listen to books on tape. If you pedal a stationary bicycle, you can read while you exercise.

Find one or more friends—especially a role model who is a regular exerciser—with whom to work out. On days you don't feel motivated to rise out of your easy chair and onto the jogging track or over to the health club, your exercise partner(s) can get you moving. If your activity sessions turn into social events, they can be a real source of enjoyment. If you're looking for exercise partners, recruit a family member or a co-worker, or join a health club, the YMCA, or a community center that offers exercise classes. Attending an exercise session at the same time each day will make it an essential part of your routine, as regular as your morning or evening bath or shower.

When you find yourself procrastinating, think about how good you feel when you do exercise, about the extra energy and equilibrium you have during the rest of the day, and how well you sleep at night. Reflect upon the way exercise is helping you maintain your weight, keep your cardiovascular system healthy, improve your peace of mind, and get your blood pressure under control. That might be the motivation you need to start moving.

Some people refuse to go to a health club, but are willing to incorporate physical activity into their everyday schedules; for example, by getting off the bus two miles from their ultimate destination and walking the rest of the way. On a particularly hectic day when your schedule just doesn't permit you to exercise formally, why not improvise some type of physical activity into your day or evening? Park your car six blocks from your office and walk briskly from the car to your desk. Skip the elevator and take the stairs to your floor. During your lunch hour, go for a walk rather than eating, or take a walk with a friend or family member after dinner.

Don't be hard on yourself or give up if you miss a few days or even weeks of exercise. Everyone backslides at times. Just get back on track as soon as possible. Think about how much better you feel since you've been following your exercise regimen, and make a commitment to exercise tomorrow.

AEROBICS AND RELAXATION: NATURAL COMPLEMENTS

Physical exercise and deep relaxation mutually enhance one another. The cycle of activity followed by rest is built into our biological rhythm. For instance:

Our activity during waking hours is naturally followed by sleep.
The active part of our breathing cycle (inhalation) is naturally followed by the relaxation part (exhalation).
The systolic (or contraction) phase of the heart's activity is followed by the diastolic phase when the heart is at rest.

Many HART patients like to relax deeply for 20 to 30 minutes before or after physical exercise. Some prefer to do their 30-minute relaxation directly before their aerobics—this enables them to re-energize prior to their exercise; others like the spontaneous deepening of their relaxation that occurs when it follows exertion. Nearly everyone has reported that exercise and relaxation are natural complements, each enhancing the other. Experiment with your own sequencing and let your own experience guide you toward what works best for you.

USE IMAGERY TO INCREASE EXERCISE'S BENEFITS

In the chapter of imagery, do you remember the report on the fitness level of the Olympic athletes? Just as imagery significantly increased their performance, taking a few extra minutes to imagine yourself enjoying and vividly engaging in your own exercise program can help increase your enjoyment, endurance, and expertise in your activity of choice. Right before you exercise, focusing briefly on the positive image you have created can be a real boost to your fitness session.

Your attitude is important when you exercise. On occasion, for example, you may arrive at your exercise class or begin a walk or other activity somewhat tired. However, by briefly relaxing and visualizing yourself vigorously and energetically enjoying aerobics, you will rapidly improve your attitude and gain new energy, enabling you to rebound and sail through the session.

If you notice your enthusiasm or enjoyment declining, picture yourself effortlessly hiking or jogging, as if you had wings on your feet. Also, inwardly affirm the way you want to feel as you move. At your exercise class, you might say, "The more I move, the more energy I feel." If you're walking or jogging: "With each stride I take, I feel better and better." For swimming: "Each stroke takes me closer to my goal."

Both the imaging and the affirmations will become blueprints for the actual exercise sessions. The more vivid you make them, the more they will enhance your enjoyment of your fitness program.

Thus, even if you haven't been physically active in years, you can choose to make regular exercise a part of your life. For example, Mark entered the HART Program with his blood pressure out of control, even though he was under a cardiologist's care and taking several antihypertensive medications. While he had practiced meditation for many years, it wasn't enough. His blood pressure was 195/110. He needed something more.

In reviewing Mark's blood pressure records at weekly sessions, it became evident that on the days he exercised, his pressure would consistently be lower than on the days he didn't work out. I encouraged him to check with his physician and to adopt a more regular exercise program. So at age 62, that's just what he did—with amazing results. From being an erratic exerciser, he began running regularly, an activity he finds particularly pleasurable. Within months, he increased his running distance so dramatically and with such enthusiasm that he started participating in 10-kilometer races—and winning trophies in his age category. Best of all, in combination with the HART Program's relaxation training, his running was having a significantly positive effect on his hypertension. On days when he found time for both exercise and relaxation periods, his blood pressure readings were lowest. At last check, a year after going through the program, his blood pressure averaged 110/70.

Incidentally, one of the best parts of working out for Mark was the people he met while exercising. He particularly valued the 80- and 90-year-olds who were setting a good example for him. One of his exercise partners—an 81-year-old woman—was about to run her eighth marathon the last time I talked with Mark. "I've got some great role models," he told me.

Mark and his friends have made a commitment to stay cardiofit for life. So can you.

CHAPTER · 17

Love, Life Purpose, and Your Cardiovascular Health

If I am not for myself, then who will be for me? If I am only for myself, then why am I here? And if not now, when?

—HILLEL THE ELDER
1st century A.D.

And now these three remain; faith, hope and love. But the greatest of these is love.

—PAUL, 1 CORINTHIANS
1st century A.D.

The truth is: love heals.

—BERNIE SIEGEL, M.D.

BY NOW, IF YOU have been applying the biobehavioral and lifestyle methods of the HART Program, you have probably already experienced significant declines in your blood pressure readings and/or medication usage, and are on the way to normalizing your blood pressure. In the process, your overall health and well-being have improved, increasing your chances for living a longer life. Blood pressure and lifestyle, while key factors in health, are not the sole determinants of quality of life and longevity.

Intuitively, many people sense that love, caring, life satisfaction, and purpose are essential to good health. Now, a growing number of studies is lending scientific credence to that premise, even suggesting how these factors may influence our physiology. Although you certainly would not have chosen to have hypertension or any other illness, you can use this disorder as an opportunity to step back, evaluate your circumstances, adjust your priorities, and along the way, free the inner physician that can help improve both your blood pressure and your life in general.

FRIENDS AS GOOD MEDICINE

The small size and isolation of the nuclear family, the prevalence of dual careers, the high rate of divorce and single-parent households, compounded by the increasing mobility in our culture and the isolation of the elderly, mean that loneliness is a major problem in the lives of many individuals. Too many people live with too little social support. They may not know their neighbors or have even a single individual they can reach out to in times of need.

Many researchers now concur that the presence or absence of social support, and the quality of the relationships we have, can be significant factors in determining how frequently we become sick and how rapidly we recover.

Consider the results of a study conducted in Alameda County, California, which not only looked at illnesses, death, and lifestyle habits (exercise, nutrition, smoking), but also the social ties of the participants in the research. The study concluded that those people who had many social connections—including marriage partners, relatives, friends, and contacts within their community and place-of-worship—had a death rate one-third to one-half the mortality among people of the same age group with few social ties. The individuals with social support lived longer and had a lower incidence of death from heart disease and other illnesses.

Additional studies have added to the evidence supporting an association between social support and good health. In Israel, for example, 10,000 civil servants were asked about both their physical ailments and their social support network. Researchers found that men who perceived their wives as loving had about one-half the incidence of angina (chest pain) as men who felt their wives were uncaring. Also, the rates of hypertension and high cholesterol were lower among those men who believed they had supportive spouses.

Even seemingly simple and ordinary efforts at reaching out to another person can make a physiological difference. Dr. James Lynch of the University of Maryland found that human touch had a positive effect on patients in the coronary care unit. He reported that when a doctor or nurse touched these patients briefly—just long enough to measure their pulse—there was a significant decline in their irregular heartbeats (ventricular arrhythmias).

The experience of the residents of Roseto, Pennsylvania, is one of the most striking examples of the influence of social connectedness on health. Roseto was a closely-knit, rural, Italian-American community that, in the 1960s, had a much lower rate of serious illnesses (including coronary heart disease and ulcers) than other cities. Doctors were initially confused by the health of the residents of Roseto, particularly since they tended to have many of the risk factors associated with heart disease, such as a high-fat diet and a relatively high incidence of hypertension and obesity.

Eventually, researchers concluded that the close, secure, social ties in Roseto were making the difference. As one health official observed, "We found that family relationships were extremely close and mutually supportive. This cohesive quality extended to neighbors and to the community as a whole."

Eventually, however, Roseto went the way of many other American cities. Roseto's younger adults, striving for more material goods and job advancements than their elders, rejected many of the traditional values that had been a part of their community for decades. Cultural ties were forgotten, family connections became less important. As these changes occurred, the death rate from heart attacks increased significantly in Roseto, particularly among middle-aged men. Researchers blamed the disintegration of the family unit and the community at large for this change in the health status of Roseto's residents.

Strengthening your social network could have significant health benefits. In one study, individuals with hypertension participated in a program designed to improve their connections with family members who could support them in their efforts to lower their blood pressure. Family and group counseling, as well as educational sessions, were designed to help hypertensives adhere to their treatment plan.

After five years, these efforts had proven worthwhile: Individuals who received social support had better blood pressure readings, lower weight, and a 57 percent lower mortality rate than people who did not receive this kind of support.

What mechanisms are at work in the protectiveness provided by human relationships? In *The Healing Brain*, Dr.'s Robert Ornstein and David Sobel wrote, "Social support and a consistent set of beliefs may work their wonders in promoting health by embedding one solidly within a fabric of stable actions and reactions to many different situations; this cushions any shock or stress and thereby prevents it from being too seriously disturbing. If the cardiovascular system is really a mirror of the mind and emotions, one who has established long-term, stable social relations and a stable place in the world has a little extra cardiovascular stability as well."

Take a moment to reflect upon your own social situation. Are there caring friends and/or family members in your life, or are you more isolated than you want to be? Could you benefit from developing closer, more supportive relationships with the people in your life, and from reaching out to develop new friendships?

THE QUALITY OF RELATIONSHIPS COUNTS

Is their someone in your life you can count on for support and in whom you can confide your innermost thoughts? Too many people answer no to this question. They may have many superficial friendships, but not the one or two special relationships where genuine sharing takes place that can contribute to their sense of living in a supportive world.

At the University of New Mexico School of Medicine, more than 250 elderly individuals participated in a study which evaluated the intimacy and intensity of their relationships. Researchers concluded that people who had strong, open friendships also possessed a number of physical characteristics (including low cholesterol, and low uric acid levels) linked with reduced rates of heart disease.

Excessive self-involvement, which precludes caring and commitment to others, can also increase cardiovascular risk. This is a real hazard in our culture, which encourages individualism rather than commitment to a larger group, be it the family, community, nation, or planet. People who are extremely self-centered—who use words like "I," "me," and "mine" throughout their conversations to the exclusion of "we" and "our"—may be setting themselves up for a socially-isolated lifestyle and some serious health consequences. These individuals may have difficulty developing or maintaining the intimate, committed relationships that could help protect them against disease.

The Multiple Risk Factor Intervention Trial (MRFIT) showed that people who died from heart attacks tended to be more self-involved than those who recovered from their coronaries. Another study, conducted by Dr. Larry Scherwitz and his associates, interviewed men with heart disease who were scheduled for coronary angiograms; those patients who were self-centered tended to have more serious coronary artery disease and a greater likelihood of having had a heart attack.

What are some sources of social support? In recent years, many thousands of people have benefited from self-help groups where they have been able to connect with other individuals facing similar challenges or sharing the same problems or illnesses. Many hypertensive patients have reported the value of participating in the HART Program with other individuals who had the same health concerns, with whom they could share their experiences and insights and give and receive support.

It may take some persistent investigation to find the support group that will best meet your needs. Check with local community centers, religious groups, counseling services, senior programs, hospitals, and event listings in your area. Also, the National Self-Help Clearinghouse (25 W. 43rd St., Room 620, New York, NY 10036) may be able to refer you to a group nearby.

LIFE SATISFACTION AND LONGEVITY

In the past, you may have been told that the path to good health was dependent on prescription pills that could lower your blood pressure, your cholesterol, or your pulse rate. In this book, however, you have had a chance to survey and hopefully make use of a fuller spectrum of resources that enable you to take charge of your blood pressure and your cardiovascular health. One of the most important of these resources is living well, during both work and leisure time.

If you feel positively about your life and your purpose, you are much more likely to be healthier and live longer than if you are depressed and disappointed with the course of your day-to-day existence. Rene Dubos, a microbiologist at Rockefeller University, studied people who had reached their 100th birthday and beyond, and concluded that their positive attitude was the most powerful characteristic they shared, even more influential than heredity or lifestyle. According to Dubos, "All of them possessed a certain eagerness to live, a certain drive, a certain general happiness."

Dr. Suzanne Kobasa, a social psychologist at the University of Chicago, analyzed the health status of high-stressed employees at AT&T, trying to determine why some stayed healthy while others fell victim to illness. She concluded that the healthy employees demonstrated three common characteristics—a feeling of *control* over their lives; a high level of *commitment* to relationships and work; and an ability to thrive in challenging circumstances.

No matter what your current situation, you can work with your inner attitude. Some of the most significant research in this field was conducted with survivors of World War II concentration camps. Psychiatrist Viktor Frankl, a camp survivor, has written about how, through a shift in attitude, he was able to psychologically elevate himself from the depths of despair, despite the horrific conditions he was forced to endure. Many of those who survived the camps made the conscious decision to perceive their experience as an opportunity to demonstrate their courage and their capacity to persevere and care for others. Despite the nightmare they were living, they refused to relinquish control over their **inner** selves.

Even in the most difficult periods of their lives, many people have shown an immense capacity and spirit for rising to the challenges life brings through a commitment to finding meaning in their present and to trusting in and working for a better future. By genuinely finding purpose in your own present, and expecting and anticipating a more promising future, you will probably not only feel healthier, you may even be adding to your own life span.

Toward that end, if you feel you could benefit from more joy in your daily life, you may wish to make a list of the activities that bring positive energy and meaning into your life. Perhaps they include listening to music, playing an instrument, gardening, biking, or hiking. Or maybe your list consists of taking friends or family to the countryside, or to plays, concerts, or museums. Also, consider activities that bring you in contact with others who share similar interests or social vision. The opportunities are boundless: participating in a reading group or a single-parent group, teaching someone to read, joining a walking club, singing in a choir, or working with groups committed to protecting our environment or bringing about needed social change.

One of the best ways to expand your social network and develop good friendships is through meeting and working with others who share interests close to your heart. Finding time for those people and commitments that nourish your well-being and fill you with positive energy will add to your life satisfaction. You will assume greater charge of your life and increase your sense of control and commitment.

By making changes in your life in favor of your health and well-being you have a greater likelihood of enjoying a life free of hypertension and other chronic illnesses. As John Knowles, former president of the Rockefeller Foundation, predicted, "The next major advance in the health of the American people will result only from what the individual is willing to do for himself."

HE WHO LAUGHS, LASTS

Dr. William Osler, a renowned Johns Hopkins Hospital physician, referred to laughter as "the music of life." Without question, laughter is another way to nurture yourself and take back more control over your well-being. By doing so, you will raise the quality of your life and augment your own self-healing.

Norman Cousins' descriptions of his own use of laughter when battling a crippling disease have been well-publicized; Cousins said that by laughing his way through old Marx Brothers movies and "Candid Camera" episodes, he experienced "an anesthetic effect" that would allow him to sleep for about two hours free of pain.

When you laugh, your brain releases an array of hormones and other chemicals. Some researchers believe that one of these substances is endorphin, a natural opiate that can ease pain and cause a euphoric feeling.

A truly "hearty" laugh can have a positive effect on the entire cardiovascular system, too, increasing the pulse rate, elevating the amount of oxygen in the blood, and giving the lungs a workout. After a hearty laugh, blood pressure and pulse rate drop below pre-laugh levels. Research at the University of California at Santa Barbara found that laughter was an excellent antidote to stress—requiring no special equipment, except for a funny bone!

THE POWER OF LOVE

How many of us feel we have realized our full potential for giving and receiving love? In the demanding pace of our lives, it is too easy to lose sight of the importance of love and caring to our health, happiness and well-being. Yet as humans, we have an innate need to feel loved and give love. If love is not part of our lives, we can experience loneliness, bitterness, anger, excessive self-involvement, and sometimes illness. Researchers now believe that love—including a healthy self-love—can augment the healing process. Unfortunately, when our hearts become emotionally bruised, there is a tendency to stop liking ourselves and to withdraw from others.

Studies have shown that when people are able to demonstrate love for others, their bodies release decreased amounts of norepinephrine, a stress hormone. Babies in orphanages who have been denied love and human touch often suffer from the "failure to thrive" syndrome, in which they never grow at normal rates; in some cases, their spines compress, they curl into a fetal-like position, and their very lives are threatened.

Research shows that when people live by themselves—without people, pets, or even plants—they have a greater incidence of coronary heart disease. One study found that when people talk to or pet their animals, their blood pressure actually declines. Pets not only provide companionship, they are also a wonderful source of love. One year after experiencing a heart attack, individuals with pets had a death rate one-fifth that of people who didn't have pets. While many people in our culture are reticent about expressing love and caring for others, our own capacity for love is unlimited and increases as it is shared.

OUR INNER SOURCE OF LOVE

Even if we have shut down in response to difficult or disappointing circumstances it is still possible to open up again, care for ourselves, and establish loving friendships and close relationships. Several years ago, I worked with a client named Daniel, who was in his middle thirties and completing work on his doctorate. Despite his academic achievements, Daniel had become cut off from healthy self-love.

Seven years earlier, Daniel had experienced a traumatic breakup with a woman he had hoped to marry; since then, he had not been willing to risk a close and intimate relationship. Even though he clearly wanted to work this problem out, he was unable to take the initiative to even ask a woman out.

From our early sessions, it became clear that Daniel needed to work on his relationship with himself before he was ready to open up to the possibility of a close relationship with a woman. He needed to develop his ability to love himself; only then could he reach out to someone else.

Daniel was very good at imaging, and part of each session would include imagery work relevant to his concerns. Together, we worked on devoting part of his imaging work to finding Daniel's inner source of love. With this goal in mind, Daniel's first image was of a hard, un-yielding, black pavement that stretched for miles. He then saw a small, dirty, muddy pool of water in an indentation in the asphalt. Daniel wondered in despair if that was all there really was.

Suddenly, the blacktop began breaking up. Beneath it was a virgin forest. Sunlight was streaming down through the fresh, green, leafy trees and a fresh bubbling stream was running through the center of the forest. A young hunter appeared, walking along the stream. Daniel had found the deeper stream of love within himself.

A short time later, Daniel met someone he cared for and they began to date. He then found an excellent teaching position, and about a year later, called to announce that he was happily married.

THE IMPORTANCE OF CONTENTMENT

Since none of us will live forever, it is important to find contentment in the context of each day—rather than waiting to be happy once we finish the next project, get a high-paying position, find the right relationship, solve the latest crisis, or lose ten pounds. Too often, we place our life satisfaction on a contingency plan, where contentment is always in the past or future, never in the present.

RE-ENVISIONING A PRESENT AND FUTURE WITH HEART

As you plan your own present and future, the following may help clarify what is really important to you. If you were told you had only a short time to live, how would you be living each day? Would your commitments be different than they are now? How would it be possible for you to devote at least part of every day—beginning now—to some of what is most important to you?

Mother Teresa is a perfect example of someone who has charted out meaning in her own life by reaching out to and serving others in need. As these words are written, Mother Teresa's own heart is almost worn out physiologically. Yet she is continuing to care and to love, and that powerful energy has overcome her physical limitations and allowed her to serve and inspire others to not only undertake great acts of love, but also to place great love within small acts.

Albert Einstein once received a letter from a rabbi who was extremely distressed by the death of his 16-year-old daughter and his inability to comfort his other child, an 18-year-old girl. Einstein responded with a moving description of how individuals fit into a larger, overall plan. He wrote:

> "A human being is part of the whole, called by us 'Universe,' a part limited in time and space. He experiences himself, his thoughts and feelings as something separate from the rest—a kind of optical delusion of his consciousness. This delusion is a kind of prison for us, restricting us to our personal desires and to affection for a few persons nearest us. Our task must be to free ourselves from this prison by widening our circle of compassion to embrace all living creatures and the whole of nature in its beauty. Nobody is able to achieve this completely, but the striving for such achievement is in itself a part of the liberation and a foundation for inner security."

Love—both a healthy self-love as well as love for others—is integral to our health and happiness. Feeling loved and actively expressing love and caring opens our heart. The open heart is the healthier heart . . . physically, spiritually, and interpersonally.

Most of us would admit that we could benefit from more love in our lives. Reaching out to build loving, supportive relationships with others is part of creating a loving life. Yet paradoxically, if we rely soley on external sources, love can often seem in short supply. By developing our own inner awareness of being loved, as well as experiencing ourselves as a radiant source of love and caring, we create the experience of a more loving and meaningful life.

The following process can create more love in our lives.

OPENING YOUR HEART

1. Sit comfortably in a balanced, symmetrical position, with your spine straight yet relaxed, and your chest open and unconstricted. Deepen your breathing and quiet your mind through practice of Three–Part Complete Breathing.
2. Close your eyes and rest your inner gaze on your heart. Focus on each cycle of breath as a balance of receiving and giving. On each "in" breath, imagine love and light flowing into your heart. On each "out" breath, see and feel love and light radiating out from you.
3. Imagine yourself sitting before the most developed, conscious, loving individual you know, someone who accepts and loves you completely and unconditionally. This can be your own wiser, higher self; someone you have met and admire; or a spiritual person to whom you feel drawn.
4. Experience this loving individual accepting and loving you completely and unconditionally. Receive this love completely.
5. Allow the love within you to flow outward to the person you imagine before you. Continue your long and deep breathing, focusing on giving and receiving love.
6. Expand your love to include those persons closest to you. Focus on each person in turn. Then expand your love to include your whole community . . . nation . . . continent . . . all the inhabitants and life on the earth and to the earth itself. Imagine the earth within your heart, and enfold it in wings of light.

Our health and happiness, the health and well-being of all those with whom we share our planet, and that of generations to come, depends on our acting on our highest visions for ourselves and humanity—with heart.

Notes

CHAPTER 1

"The patients who . . .". This quote from Dr. Patricia Norris appears in *Hypertension: A Problem of Control,* a videotape produced by the University of Illinois, 1985.

health statistics. American Heart Association, 7320 Greenville Avenue, Dallas, TX 75231.

"An elevated arterial blood pressure . . .". Robert G. Petersdorf, et al., eds., *Harrison's Principles of Internal Medicine* (McGraw-Hill Book Company, 1983).

biobehavioral treatment for hypertension. Steven L. Fahrion, Patricia A. Norris, Alyce M. Green and Elmer E. Green, "Biobehavioral Treatment of Essential Hypertension: A Group Outcome Study." In *Biofeedback and Self-Regulation* (in press); Dobbi A. Kerman, *Cost-Effective, Non-Pharmacological Biobehavioral Treatment of Essential Hypertension,* doctoral dissertation, 1986.

"Those who persist . . .". Elmer E. Green, Menninger Foundation, Topeka, KS.

CHAPTER 3

"The greatest force . . ." Norman Cousins, *Human Options* (W.W. Norton, 1981).

While blood pressure increases during exercise, the long-term result of regular aerobic activity is a stronger, more efficient heart which pumps more slowly yet with more blood per beat, during both exercise and rest. This contributes to a lower heart rate and blood pressure.

stress. Hans Selye, *The Stress of Life* (New York: McGraw-Hill, 1956); Robert S. Eliot and Dennis L. Breo, *Is It Worth Dying For?* (Bantam, 1984).

Holmes-Rahe scale. Thomas H. Holmes and Richard H. Rahe, "The Social Readjustment Rating Scale," *Journal of Psychomatic Research,* 11:213–18, 1967.

"The way we perceive . . ." Robert Ornstein and David Sobel, *The Healing Brain* (Simon & Schuster, 1987).

thrive on stress. Kenneth Pelletier, *Mind as Healer, Mind as Slayer* (Dell, 1977).

stress and the spice of life. Elmer Green and Alyce Green, "General and Specific Applications of Thermal Biofeedback," from *Biofeedback: Principles and Practice for Clinicians,* John V. Basmajian (ed.), 1st edition (Williams & Wilkins Co., 1979).

stress, job pressure and urban anxiety. R.M. Jenkins, et al., "Air Traffic Controller Health Change Study: A Prospective Investigation of Physical, Psychological and Work-Related Changes" (Contract No. DOT-FA737WA-3211), Boston University School of Medicine, 1978; Blair Justice, *Who Gets Sick* (Jeremy P. Tarcher, Inc., 1988).

hot reacting and blood pressure. Eliot and Breo, *Is It Worth Dying For?*

"When the mind receives. . . ." Barbara Brown, *Stress and the Art of Biofeedback* (Harper & Row, 1977).

biofeedback case study. Elmer E. Green, Alyce M. Green, Patricia A. Norris, "Self-Regulation Training for Control of Hypertension," *Primary Cardiology,* 6:126–137, 1980.

when feedback indicates decreases in sympathetic nervous system activity. Stimulating the sympathetic branch of the ANS (Autonomic Nervous System) increases blood pressure, while decreasing the activity of the sympathetic system lowers blood pressure.

early feedback research. Chandra Patel, "Yoga and Biofeedback in the Management of Hypertension," *Lancet,* 2:1053–1055, 1973; Chandra Patel, "Biofeedback-Aided Relaxation and Mediation in the Management of Hypertension," *Biofeedback and Self-Regulation,* 2;1–41, 1977; Chandra Patel and M. Carruthers, "Coronary Risk Factor Reduction Through Biofeedback-Aided Relaxation and Meditation, *Journal of the Royal College of General Practice,* 27:401–405, 1977.

Menninger research. Elmer Green, et al., "Self-Regulation Training for Control of Hypertension."

Biofeedback and high blood pressure. Keith Sedlack, et al., "Comparison Between Biofeedback and Relaxation Response in the Treatment of Essential Hypertension," *Proceedings,* Biofeedback Society of America, 1979, p. 84–87; Edward Blanchard et al., "A Comparison of Thermal Biofeedback and Autogenic Training in the Treatment of Mild Hypertension: Preliminary Findings," *Proceedings,* Biofeedback Society of America, 1986, p. 23–25; M. Hartfield, "Effects of a Self-Regulation Model on Reducing Hypertension," *Proceedings,* Biofeedback Society of America, 1986, p. 49–51.

CHAPTER 4

stepped care/step zero. "Joint National Committee on Detection, Evaluation, and Treatment of High Blood Pressure: The 1984 Report," *Archives of Internal Medicine,* 144:1045–1057, 1984.

drug side effects. Norman M. Kaplan, *Clinical Hypertension,* 4th edition (Williams & Wilkins Co., 1986); J.D. Curb, et al., "Long-Term Surveillance for Adverse Effects of Antihypertensive Drugs," *Journal of the American Medical Association,* 253:3264–68, 1985; William Stason and Milton Weinstein, "Public Health Records of the Harvard School of Public Health: Allocation of Resources to Manage Hypertension," *New England Journal of Medicine,* 296: 732–739, 1977.

treatment of hypertension. Douglas Gasner and Elliott H. McClery, *The AMA Book of Heart Care* (Random House, 1982).

adherence to treatment. "Joint National Committee on Detection, Evaluation, and Treatment of High Blood Pressure."

choosing a physician. Herbert Benson, *The Relaxation Response* (William Morrow, 1975).

CHAPTER 5

"We do know . . .". This quote from Edward Lichter, M.D., appears in *Hypertension: A Problem of Control,* a videotape produced by the University of Illinois, Chicago, 1985.

"Nonpharmacologic intervention . . .". Rose Stamler and Jeremiah Stamler, " 'Mild' Hypertension: Risks and Strategy," *Primary Cardiology,* 9:150–166, 1983.

redefinition of hypertension. "Joint National Committee on Detection, Evaluation, and Treatment of High Blood Pressure."

blood pressure goals. Norman Kaplan, "Hypertension." In: *Prevention of Coronary Heart Disease,* Norman Kaplan and Jeremiah Stamler, eds. (W.B. Saunders Co., 1983); Stamler and Stamler, " 'Mild' Hypertension: Risks and Strategy."

actuarial data. American Heart Association, 7320 Greenville Ave., Dallas, TX 75231

"The higher the blood pressure . . .". Kaplan, "Hypertension." In: *Prevention of Coronary Heart Disease.*

world statistics. World Health Organization, Avenue Appia, CH-1211, Geneva 27, Switzerland.

risk factors. Eliot and Breo, *Is It Worth Dying For?*

CHAPTER 6

measuring blood pressure. Some controversy still exists about when to measure the diastolic pressure. Although some doctors believe it should be assessed when a final muffled noise is heard just before the disappearance of all sound (phase 4 of the so-called Korotkoff's sounds), they are in the minority. Current recommendations for calculating adult blood pressure advise recording the diastolic pressure when silence occurs (phase 5). In children, however, because their cardiac output is high, sounds can often be heard throughout the deflation of the cuff; thus, diastolic pressure is measured during the final, faint, swishing sound (phase 4).

use of the wrong sized cuff. David S. Sobel and Tom Ferguson, *The People's Book of Medical Tests* (Summit Books, 1985).

blood pressure equipment. All of the original blood pressure measuring equipment incorporated a graduated glass cylinder that contained mercury. In keeping with this standard of measurement, blood pressure is still measured in "millimeters of mercury" today, even though many of our current devices actually contain no mercury.

formula for blood pressure. The volume of blood expelled by the heart is equal to the amount of blood ejected at each beat multiplied by the number of beats within a given time interval.

CHAPTER 7

self-regulatory capacity. Brown, *Stress and the Art of Biofeedback.*

CHAPTER 8

reverse breathers. Dobbi A. Kerman, Patricia A. Norris, Steven L. Fahrion, *HART: Hypertension, Autonomic, Relaxation Treatment, Clinical Manual for the Bio-Behavioral Treatment of High Blood Pressure,* 1984.

CHAPTER 9

"If you relax . . .". Edmund Jacobson, *You Must Relax* (McGraw-Hill Book Company, 1976).

"[I]n most kinds . . ." and *"If muscles are not . . .".* Brown, *Stress and the Art of Biofeedback.*

Jacobson's research. Jacobson, *You Must Relax.*

forcing yourself to relax. David Bresler and Richard Trubo, *Free Yourself from Pain* (Simon & Schuster, 1979).

"The time to relax . . .". This Sidney Harris quote is cited in Dean Ornish. *Stress, Diet and Your Heart* (Holt, Rinehart & Winston, 1982).

CHAPTER 10

power of imagery. Robert Swearingen, "Meditation in the Emergency Room," in *Body, Mind and Health: Toward an Integral Medicine* (J. Gordon, D. Jaffe and D. Bresler, eds.), National Institute of Mental Health Monograph, 1980.

capable of increasing blood flow. Norman Cousins, *Head First* (E.P. Dutton, 1989).

Dr. Ornish's research. Ornish, *Stress, Diet and Your Heart.*

Simonton's research. O. Carl Simonton, Stephanie Matthews-Simonton, and James Creighton, *Getting Well Again* (J.P. Tarcher, 1978).

Pribram/Soviet studies. For a discussion of Karl Pibram's research, and studies of Soviet athletes, see Charles Garfield, *Peak Performance* (Jeremy P. Tarcher, 1984).

CHAPTER 11

stress and hypertension. Eliot and Breo, *Is It Worth Dying For?*

Patel's research. Chandra Patel, et al., "Randomised Controlled Trial of Yoga and Biofeedback in Management of Hypertension," *Lancet* 2:93–95, p. 93–95.

"island of peace." Pelletier, *Mind as Healer, Mind as Slayer.*

Yerkes-Dodson Law. Kenneth R. Pelletier, *Healthy People in Unhealthy Places* (Delacorte Press, 1984).

"Just about anybody . . .". This Clifford Odets quote came from the 1954 motion picture adaptation of his play, *The Country Girl.*

"The harder things get . . .". This quote, appearing as number 10 on the list on page 137, is by Boris N. Yeltsin, quoted in the *New York Times,* August 26, 1991, p. A6.

"Rule No. 1 . . .". Eliot and Breo, *Is It Worth Dying For?*

"grant me the courage . . .". from "The Serenity Prayer," a sermon delivered by Reinhold Niebuhr at the Congregational church of Heath, Mass.

CHAPTER 12

"If you are among . . .". C. Everett Koop, as quoted in Warren E. Leary, "Major U.S. Report on the Diet Urges Reduction in Fat Intake," *New York Times,* January 28, 1988, p. 1.

"A high intake . . .". William B. Kannel, "Diet, Serum Cholesterol, Lipoproteins, and Coronary Heart Disease." In: *Prevention of Coronary Heart Disease,* Norman Kaplan and Jeremiah Stamler, eds. (W.B. Saunders Co., 1983).

low-fat diets. J.M. Iacono, et al., "Reduction of Blood Pressure Associated with High Polyunsaturated Fat Diets That Reduce Blood Cholesterol in Man," *Preventive Medicine,* 4:426–443, 1975; P. Puska, et al., "Controlled, Randomized Trial of the Effect of Dietary Fat on Blood Pressure," *Lancet,* 1:1–15, 1983.

cholesterol and heart disease. National Cholesterol Education Program, *Report of the Expert Panel on Detection, Evaluation and Treatment of High Blood Cholesterol in Adults,* National Institutes of Health Publication No. 88–2925, 1988.

fish and cardiovascular health. Daan Kromhout, et al., "The Inverse Relation Between Fish Consumption and 20-Year Mortality from Coronary Heart Disease, *New England Journal of Medicine,* 312:1205–1209, 1985; Howard R. Knapp and Garret A. FitzGerald, "The Antihypertensive Effects of Fish Oil," *New England Journal of Medicine,* 320:1037–1043, 1989; and P. G. Norris, et al., "Effect of Dietary Supplementation with Fish Oil in Systolic Blood Pressure in Mild Essential Hypertension," *British Medical Journal,* 293:104–105, 1986.

complex carbohydrates. Daan Kromhout, et al., "Dietary Fibre and 10-Year Mortality From CHD, Cancer and All Causes," *Lancet,* 2:518–521, 1982; Judith J. Wurtman, "The Involvement of Brain Serotonin in Excessive Carbohydrate Snacking By Obese Carbohydrate Cravers," *Journal of the American Dietetic Association,* 84:1004–1007, 1984; and Richard Wurtman, "Behavioural Effects of Nutrients," *Lancet,* 1:1145–1147, 1983.

fiber and blood pressure. A. Wright, et al., "Dietary Fibre and Blood Pressure," *British Medical Journal,* 2:1541–1543, 1979; James W. Anderson, "Plant Fiber and Blood Pressure," *Annals of Internal Medicine,* 98:842–846, 1983.

sugar and hypertension. Ronald S. Smith, *Nutrition, Hypertension & Cardiovascular Disease* (Lyncean Press, 1989).

garlic and hypertension. A. Bordia, et al., "Effect of Garlic on Regression of Atherosclerosis in Rabbits," *Artery,* 7:428–437, 1980; S. Barrie, et al., "Effects of Garlic Oil on Platelets, Serum Lipids and Blood Pressure in Humans," *Journal of Orthomolecular Medicine,* 2:15–21, 1987; and Smith, *Nutrition, Hypertension & Cardiovascular Disease.*

coffee and hypertension. H. Ammon, et al., "Adaption of Blood Pressure to Heavy Coffee Drinking," *British Journal of Clinical Pharmacology,* 15:701–706, 1983.

alcohol and hypertension. Intersalt Cooperative Research Group, "Intersalt: An International Study," *British Medical Journal,* 297:319–328,

1988; Charles H. Hennekens, "Alcohol." In: *Prevention of Coronary Heart Disease*, Norman Kaplan and Jeremiah Stamler, eds. (W. B. Saunders Co., 1983); S. MacMahon, et al., "Obesity, Alcohol Consumption and Blood Pressure in Australian Men and Women: The National Heart Foundation of Australia Risk Factor Prevalence Study," *Journal of Hypertension*, 2:85–91, 1984; and Smith, *Nutrition, Hypertension & Cardiovascular Disease.*

"The three most common . . .". Frances Moore Lappe, *Diet for a Small Planet* (Ballantine Books, 1982).

Ornish research. Dean Ornish, *Dr. Dean Ornish's Program for Reversing Heart Disease* (Random House, 1990).

CHAPTER 13

"Dietary potassium, calcium . . .". Rose Stamler and Jeremiah Stamler, " 'Mild' Hypertension: Risks and Strategy," *Primary Cardiology* 9:150–166, 1983.

mechanisms of sodium. Norman M. Kaplan, *Clinical Hypertension* (Williams & Wilkins, 1986); Norman M. Kaplan, *Management of Hypertension* (Creative Infomatics, 1987).

sodium and hypertension. U.S. Department of Health and Human Services, *The Surgeon General's Report on Nutrition & Health* (Warner Books, 1989); Smith, *Nutrition, Hypertension & Cardiovascular Disease;* James Hunt, "Sodium Intake and Hypertension: A Cause for Concern," *Annals of Internal Medicine*, 98:724, 1983; James J. Nora, *The Whole Heart Book* (Holt, Rinehart & Winston, 1980); Adele Davis, *Let's Get Well* (Harcourt, Brace, Javonovich, 1965); J. Sullivan, et al., "Sodium Sensitivity in Normotensive and Borderline Hypertensive Humans," *American Journal of Medical Science*, 295:370–377, 1988; Australian National Health and Medical Research Council Dietary Salt Study Management Committee, "Fall in Blood Pressure with Modest Reduction in Dietary Salt Intake in Mild Hypertension," *Lancet*, 1:399–402, 1989; G.D. Bompiani, et al., "Effects of Moderate Low Sodium/High Potassium Diet on Essential Hypertension: Results of a Comparative Study," *International Journal of Clinical Pharmacology, Therapy & Toxicology*, 26:129–132, 1988; Jeremiah Stamler, et al., "Prevention and Control of Hypertension by Nutritional-Hygienic Means," *Journal of the American Medical Association*, 243:1819–1823, 1980.

potassium and high blood pressure. H. Langford, "Dietary Potassium and Hypertension: Epidemiological Data," *Annals of Internal Medicine*, 98:770–772, 1983; and K. Khaw, et al., "Dietary Potassium and Stroke-Associated Mortality," *New England Journal of Medicine*, 316:235–240, 1987.

calcium and hypertension. David McCarron, et al., "Blood Pressure and Nutrient Intake in the United States," *Science,* 224:1392–1398, 1984; David McCarron, "Calcium and Magnesium Nutrition in Human Hypertension," *Annals of Internal Medicine,* 98:800–805, 1983; David McCarron, et al., "Blood Pressure Response to Oral Calcium," *Annals of Internal Medicine,* 103:825–831, 1985; Nancy Johnson, et al., "Effects on Blood Pressure of Calcium Supplementation of Women," *American Journal of Clinical Nutrition,* 42:12–17, 1985.

magnesium and high blood pressure. Smith, *Nutrition, Hypertension & Cardiovascular Disease;* M. Joffres, et al., "Magnesium Intake and Blood Pressure: Honolulu Heart Study," *American Journal of Clinical Nutrition,* 45:468–475, 1987; Thomas Dyckner, et al., "Effect of Magnesium on Blood Pressure," *British Medical Journal,* 286:1847–1849, 1983; William Mroczek, et al., "Effect of Magnesium Sulfate on Cardiovascular Hemodynamics," *Angiology,* 28:720–724, 1977; W. Davis, et al., "Effect of Oral Magnesium Chloride on the QT and QU Intervals of the EKG," *South African Medical Journal,* 53:591–593, 1978; Thomas Dyckner, et al., "Effects of Magnesium Infusions in Diuretic Induced Hyponatraemia," *Lancet,* 1:585–586, 1981; and I. Dorup, et al., "Reduced Concentration of Potassium, Magnesium and Sodium-Potassium Pumps in Skeletal Muscle Using Diuretics," *British Medical Journal,* 296:455–458, 1988.

chromium and hypertension. W. Mertz, "Chromium Occurrence and Function in Biological Systems," *Physiological Reviews,* 49:163–239, 1969; and Smith, *Nutrition, Hypertension & Cardiovascular Disease.*

vitamin C and heart disease. Smith, *Nutrition, Hypertension & Cardiovascular Disease;* and Emil Ginter, "Pretreatment Serum Cholesterol and Response to Ascorbic Acid," *Lancet,* 2:958–959, 1979.

vitamin E. William Hermann, "The Effect of Vitamin E on Lipoprotein Cholesterol Distribution," *Annals of the New York Academy of Sciences,* 393:467–472, 1982.

selenium. Smith, *Nutrition, Hypertension & Cardiovascular Disease.*

niacin. Peter Kwiterovich, *Beyond Cholesterol: The Johns Hopkins Complete Guide for Avoiding Heart Disease* (Johns Hopkins University Press, 1989); and David Blakenhorn, et al., "Beneficial Effects of Combined Colestipol-Niacin Therapy on Coronary Atherosclerosis and Coronary Venous Bypass Grafts," *Journal of the American Medical Association,* 257:3233–3240, 1987.

vitamin B6. J. Rinehart, "Vitamin B6 Deficiency in the Rhesus Monkey with Particular Reference to the Occurrence of Atherosclerosis," *American Journal of Clinical Nutrition,* 4:318–328, 1956.

vitamin D. S. Taura, et al., "Vitamin D-Induced Coronary Atherosclerosis in Normolipemic Swine," *Tohoku Journal of Experimental Medicine,* 129:9–16, 1979.

CHAPTER 14

"We have evidence . . .". Kaplan, "Hypertension." In: *Prevention of Coronary Heart Disease*.

distribution of body fat. Richard P. Donahue, et al., "Central Obesity and Coronary Heart Disease in Men," *Lancet*, 8537:821–824, 1987. To get a good indication of your own body fat status, calculate your waist-to-hip ratio. For instance, if your waist measures 33 inches and your hips measure 39 inches, your ratio is .84 (33 divided by 39 = .84). According to researchers at the Cooper Clinic in Dallas, the acceptable waist-to-hip ratio is .85 or lower [Neil F. Gordon and Larry W. Gibbons, *The Cooper Clinic Cardiac Rehabilitation Program* (Simon & Schuster, 1990)].

weight loss. F.W. Ashley, et al., "Relation of Weight Change to Changes in Atherogenic Traits: The Framingham Study," *Journal of Chronic Diseases*, 27:103–114, 1974; E. Reisin, et al., "Effect of Weight Loss without Salt Restriction on the Reduction of Blood Pressure in Overweight Hypertensive Patients," *New England Journal of Medicine*, 298:1–6, 1978; U.S. Department of Health and Human Services, *The Surgeon General's Report on Nutrition and Health*; and Gordon and Gibbons, *The Cooper Clinic Cardiac Rehabilitation Program*.

food and mood. Justice, *Who Gets Sick*.

CHAPTER 15

smoking cessation. Surgeon General Antonia C. Novello, U.S. Department of Health and Human Services, quoted in Philip J. Hilts, "Report Cities Health Gains for the Smokers Who Quit," *New York Times*, September 26, 1990, p. A12.

impact of smoking. American Heart Association, "Smoking and Heart Disease," (American Heart Association, 1987).

quitting and backsliding. U.S. Department of Health and Human Services, *The Health Benefits of Smoking Cessation* (Public Health Service, 1990); and M.C. Fiore, et al., "Methods Used to Quit Smoking in the United States: Do Cessation Programs Help?" *Journal of the American Medical Association*, 263:2760–2765, 1990.

CHAPTER 16

warnings against exercise. Cecil, R.L. (ed.), *Cecil's A Textbook of Medicine* (W.B. Saunders Co., 1927). Oglesby, Paul, "Background on the Prevention of Cardiovascular Disease," *Circulation*, 80:206–214, 1989.

"Exercise to keep fit . . .". This quote by Dr. Paul Dudley White is from an unpublished 1929 manuscript, *Heart Disease and Its Prevention*. It is part of the Paul Dudley White archive at the Countway Library of Medicine at Harvard University, Boston, MA.

aerobics. Aerobic exercise requires increased oxygen use over an extended time period (minimally fifteen minutes), and involves the continuous movement of large muscles that can speed up the flow of blood to the heart. With these exercises, individuals can work out in their target heart zone, a range required to achieve cardiovascular fitness.

cardiovascular advantages of exercise. Gordon and Gibbons, *The Cooper Clinic Cardiac Rehabilitation Program*; Kenneth Cooper, *The Aerobics Way* (M. Evans and Company, 1977); Steven Blair, et al., "Physical Fitness and Incidence of Hypertension in Healthy, Normotensive Men and Women," *Journal of the American Medical Association*, 252:487–490, 1984.

Paffenbarger research. Ralph Paffenbarger, et al., "Work Activity and Coronary Heart Disease Mortality," *New England Journal of Medicine*, 292:545–550, 1975; Ralph Paffenbarger, et al., "Physical Activity, All-Cause Mortality, and Longevity in College Alumni," *New England Journal of Medicine*, 314:605–613, 1986.

exercise/hypertension research. Blair, "Physical Fitness and the Incidence of Hypertension in Healthy Normotensive Men and Women;" Jeremiah Stamler, et al., "Prevention and Control of Hypertension by Nutritional Hygienic Means," *Journal of the American Medical Association*, 244:1819–1823, 1980; Robert Cade, et al., "Effect of Aerobic Exercise Training on Patients with Systemic Arterial Hypertension," *American Journal of Medicine*, 77:785–790, 1984; and Edward B. Blanchard, et al., *Non-Drug Treatments for Essential Hypertension* (Pergamon Press, 1988).

exercise and stress/emotional well-being. James A. Blumenthal, et al., "Effects of Exercise on the Type A (Coronary-Prone) Behavior Pattern," *Psychosomatic Medicine*, 42:289–296, 1980; Callen, K.E., "Mental and Emotional Aspects of Long-Distance Running," *Psychomatics*, 24:133–151, 1983; and R.M. Hayden, "Physical Fitness and Mental Health," paper presented at meeting of the American Psychological Association in Toronto, 1984.

benefits of walking. James M. Haberg, "Effect of Exercise Training in 60 to 69-Year-Old Persons with Essential Hypertension," *American Journal of Cardiology*, 64:348–353, 1989.

frequency of exercise. Kenneth Cooper, *The Aerobics Program for Total Well-Being* (M. Evans and Co., 1982).

perceived exercise level. Gordon and Gibbons, *The Cooper Clinic Cardiac Rehabilitation Program*.

CHAPTER 17

"The truth is . . ." Bernie Siegel, *Love, Medicine and Miracles* (Harper & Row, 1986).

social ties. Lisa Berkman, et al., "Resistance, and Mortality: A Nine-Year Follow-Up Study of Alameda County Residents," *American Journal of Epidemiology*, 109:186–204, 1979. The Israeli study is described in: J.H. Medalie and U. Goldbourt, "Angina Pectoris Among 10,000 Men, II: Psychosocial and Other Risk Factors," *American Journal of Medicine*, 60:910–921, 1976.

human touch. James J. Lynch, *The Broken Heart* (Basic Books, 1977).

Roseto residents. J. Bruhn, "An Epidemiological Study of Myocardial Infarctions in an Italian-American community," *Journal of Chronic Diseases*, 18:353–365, 1965.

advantages/benefits of social support. Ornstein and Sobel, *The Healing Brain*; D.E. Morisky, et al., "Evaluation of Family Health Education to Build Social Support for Long Term Control of High Blood Pressure," *Health Education Quarterly*, 12:35–50, 1985; Larry Scherwitz, et al., "Self-Involvement and the Risk Factors for Coronary Heart Disease," *Advances*, 2:6–18, 1985.

"Social support and . . .". Ornstein and Sobel, *The Healing Brain*.

100 birthdays and beyond. Rene Dubos, comments on *Self-Healing*, a sound recording from the Institute for the Study of Human Knowledge (Healing Brain Series Cassette Recording #15), 1981.

Suzanne C. Kobasa, "Stressful Life Events, Personality, and Health: An Inquiry Into Hardiness," *Journal of Personality and Social Psychology*, 37:1–11, 1979; Suzanne C. Kobasa, et al., "Hardiness and Health: A Prospective Study," *Journal of Personality and Social Psychology*, 42:168–77, 1982.

concentration camp survivors. Viktor Frankl, *Man's Search for Meaning*, (Beacon Press, 1962).

Knowles prediction. John Knowles was quoted in *Time*, August 6, 1976, p. 62.

"the music of life." This William Osler quote appears in Bernie Siegel, *Love, Medicine & Miracles* (Harper & Row, 1986).

laughter. Norman Cousins, *Anatomy of an Illness* (W.W. Norton & Co., 1979); "Laughing Toward Longevity," *University of California, Berkeley, Wellness Letter*, June 1985, p. 1

importance of love/effect on stress hormones. Justice, *Who Gets Sick*; Daniel Goleman, "The Experience of Touch: Research Points to a Crucial Role," *New York Times*, February 2, 1988, p. 22.

pets. Panel discussion on social support provided by pets, conducted at American Association for the Advancement of Science meeting, Pacific division, June 1984 in San Francisco.

Appendix I

TEN STEPS TO TAKING YOUR BLOOD PRESSURE

1. Sit quietly for a few minutes before taking your blood pressure. It is best to be in a quiet place, free of distractions, since you'll need to listen carefully for tapping sounds through the stethoscope.

2. Sit with your arm extended and your palm up, slightly bent, and resting comfortably on a table at about the same level as your heart. Your back should be supported by your chair. Keep your legs uncrossed and rest your feet flat on the floor. (If you assume other positions, such as sitting with your back unsupported, standing, or reclining, your measurements will probably be different than those you get while seated with your back supported.) Then bare the skin of your upper, nondominant arm, making sure that if you are wearing long sleeves, your rolled sleeve is not constricting blood flow. You should be able to place at least two fingers under your sleeve.

3. The sounds that help you determine your blood pressure come from your brachial pulse. To find it, bend your arm at the elbow, positioning your forearm at a right angle. Make a fist so your upper arm muscles bulge. Just above the center of the upper arm, you will see or feel (by gentle probing) an indentation where your bicep and tricep muscles meet. With a gentle but firm touch, using the pads of your middle and forefingers, press into that space or indentation in the belly of the muscle until you feel a pulsing. This is your brachial artery pulse. Re-

member where it is located since you will be positioning the head of your stethoscope over this point.

4. Make sure the rubber tubing is coming out of the bottom of the cuff. Wrap the cuff snugly around your upper arm so the lower edge of the cuff is just above the bend of your elbow. The cuff should be smooth, unwrinkled, and wrapped around your skin, not your clothing. If you are using a cuff with a built-in stethoscope, **the head of the stethoscope should be positioned on top of your brachial artery pulse.** If you are using a blood pressure unit with a separate stethoscope, position the cuff so it is one inch above your elbow crease.

   Place the head of the stethoscope over your brachial artery pulse firmly but lightly, so its full circumference is in contact with the skin. Keep the stethoscope head from rubbing against tubing or clothing to prevent extraneous noise.

   Adjust the pliable metal ear pieces of the stethoscope to your head size for comfort. Place the stethoscope ear pieces in your ears, with the plastic tips angled forward.

   For the next step, either hold the round gauge so you can see the dial, or, if you prefer your hands free, clip the gauge onto its box or some other support. Make sure you can look straight at the dial so you will read it more accurately.

5. Close the metal valve just below the rubber bulb by turning the valve clockwise. Don't tighten the valve so much that you have to wrestle it open, but do close it completely. Then inflate the cuff by rapidly squeezing the rubber bulb. You will be able to feel the cuff tightening. Watch the hand on the dial of the gauge as you continue increasing the pressure in the cuff. Inflate the cuff until the gauge reads approximately 30 mm Hg above your systolic pressure. For example, if your systolic pressure is usually 170 mm Hg,

raise the dial reading to 200. If you are uncertain what your systolic pressure usually is, inflate the cuff to 210.

6. Open the metal valve a little bit by turning it very slightly counterclockwise. Gradually and smoothly, adjust the valve as needed to deflate the cuff at the slow, steady rate of 2 to 3 mm Hg per second. This means you want to see the hand on the dial pulse two to three times within the two longer lines of each ten-unit increment on the gauge. Although this takes some practice, you will pick it up quickly.

7. As you continue deflating the cuff, you will soon hear the onset of clear regular tapping noises that gradually increase in intensity. When you hear the **first** of these tapping sounds, note the reading on the dial. This is your *systolic pressure*. (If you miss hearing this first beat, do not reinflate the cuff in the middle of this whole process. Instead, deflate the cuff entirely, wait about a minute, then start again.)

8. Continue to decrease the cuff pressure at the constant rate of 2 to 3 mm Hg per second. Soon, the sounds will become muffled (they may even briefly disappear), followed by the onset of loud, regular knocking sounds that gradually fade out. At the moment that all sound disappears, note the gauge reading. This is your *diastolic pressure*. Then, open the metal valve completely, allowing all remaining pressure out of the cuff and releasing the pressure on your arm. (If you miss taking a reading at the point at which all sound vanishes, do not reinflate the cuff in the midst of this process and try to take a measurement. Let all the air out of the cuff, wait a minute, then repeat the measurement process.)

9. Record your systolic and diastolic pressure. For example, if you heard the first regular beat at 125 and all sound disappeared at 85, you would record 125/85.

10. Repeat steps 5 through 9 twice. Then calculate the averages of your systolic and diastolic readings by adding all the systolic readings and dividing by the number of measurements. For example, if your systolic readings are 120, 130 and 125:

120 + 130 + 125 = 375

375   divided by   3 = 125

Enter 125 as your average systolic reading. Follow the same process to determine your average diastolic measurement. Enter these average readings in your Daily Blood Pressure log (on page 252). Remember to pause briefly between measurements to allow your circulation to return to normal. Raising the arm (with the cuff on it) above your head will rapidly restore normal circulation. It is particularly important to take three blood pressure readings using this process if your blood pressure tends to vary from reading to reading within a short time interval (labile blood pressure), or if your initial blood pressure values are higher than you had expected. When you are first learning to take your blood pressure, repeated measurements also increase your familiarity and comfort with the measurement process.

Appendix II

H.A.R.T. DAILY BLOOD PRESSURE LOG:

NAME _____

PHYSICIAN _____

Session	Date	Blood Pressure				Pulse		Temperature	
		Before		After		Before	After	Before	After
		sys	dias	sys	dias			H = hand F = foot	
Wk. Average									
Wk. Average									
Month Average									

CHARTING YOUR PROGRESS

Starting Medication	Dosage	Time

Subjective Level of Tension Relaxation -10 0 +10 Before | After	Weight	Medication Changes	Insights and Observations

H.A.R.T. CIP STRESS

CIP Strategies

1. Practice CIP hourly and more frequently in stressful situations.
2. Use cues as reminder to practice CIP.
3. Use stressful situations as opportunities to implement CIP goals.

DAY_____ DATE _____

TIME	HOURLY USE OF CIP	STRESSOR	
6:00			
7:00			
8:00			
9:00			
10:00			
11:00			
12:00			
1:00			
2:00			
3:00			
4:00			
5:00			
6:00			
7:00			
8:00			
9:00			
10:00			
11:00			
12:00			

Summary Observations:

MANAGEMENT LOG

4. Use mental rehersal to assist you in implememting CIP goals.
5. Review your goals daily, use your skills frequently. Take a few minutes each day to observe how your performance matches your goals.
6. Acknowledge/praise yourself for using CIP skills.

TEMPERATURE		SUBJECTIVE LEVEL		INSIGHTS AND OBSERVATIONS
		Tension	Relaxtion	
		-10 0	+10	
Before	After	Before	After	

© D. Ariel Kerman, HART Institute, Chicago, IL

Index

Permissions

Note: The following items have been reproduced with permission as stated below. We have carefully researched and obtained these permissions in writing. Any error or omission herein is unintentional.

Excerpt which appears on page vi from Kenneth R. Pelletier, Ph.D., *Longevity: Fulfilling Our Biological Potential.* Copyright © 1981 by Kenneth R. Pelletier, published by Delacorte Press. Reprinted by permission of the author.

Excerpt which appears on page 16 from Norman Cousins, *Human Options.* Copyright © 1981 by Norman Cousins. Reprinted by permission of the publisher, W.W. Norton & Company, Inc.

Excerpts which appear on pages 21 and 227 from Robert Ornstein and David Sobel, *The Healing Brain.* Copyright © 1987 by The Institute for the Study of Human Behavior. Reprinted by permission of the publisher, Simon & Schuster.

Excerpts which appear on pages 25, 95, and 98 from Barbara B. Brown, *Stress and the Art of Biofeedback.* Copyright © 1977 by Barbara B. Brown. Reprinted by permission of the author.

Excerpt which appears on page 35 from Herbert Benson, M.D., *Beyond the Relaxation Response.* Copyright © 1984 by Times Books. Reprinted by permission of the publisher, Times Books, a division of Random House, Inc.

Quote which appears on page 36 by Edward Lichter, M.D., from a videotape produced by the University of Illinois at Chicago (1985). Used here by permission of Dr. Lichter.

Excerpts which appear on pages 41 and 138 from Dr. Robert S. Eliot and Dennis L. Breo, *Is It Worth Dying For?* Copyright © 1984 by Robert S. Eliot, M.D., Dennis L Breo. Reprinted by permission of the publisher, Bantam Books, a division of Bantam, Doubleday, Dell Publishing Group, Inc.

Excerpt which appears on page 95 from Edmund Jacobson, *You Must Relax.* Copyright © 1976 by Edmund Jacobson. Reprinted by permission of the publisher, McGraw-Hill, Inc.

Excerpt which appears on page 108 from *Head First: The Biology of Hope* by Norman Cousins. Copyright © 1989 by Norman Cousins. Used by permission of the publisher, Dutton, an imprint of New American Library, a division of Penguin Books USA Inc.

Excerpts which appear on pages 143 and 186 from *Prevention of Coronary Heart Disease* edited by Norman M. Kaplan, M.D. and Jeremiah Stamler, M.D. Copyright © 1983 by W.B. Saunders Company. Reprinted by permission of the publisher, W.B. Saunders Company.

Chart which appears on page 153, adapted from Julian Whitaker, M.D., *Reversing*